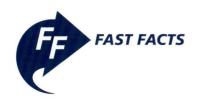 **FAST FACTS**

2
SECOND
EDITION

Multiple Myeloma and Plasma Cell Dyscrasias

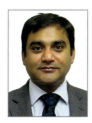

Karthik Ramasamy PhD FRCP FRCPath
Consultant Haematologist
NIHR Thames Valley and South Midlands LCRN:
Cancer Research Lead
Churchill Hospital, Oxford University Hospitals NHS Trust
Oxford, UK

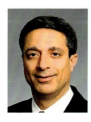

Sagar Lonial MD FACP
Professor and Chair
Department of Hematology and Medical Oncology
Chief Medical Officer, Winship Cancer Institute
Emory University
Atlanta, GA, USA

D1677503

Declaration of Independence
This book is as balanced and as practical as we can make it.
Ideas for improvement are always welcome at **fastfacts.com**

 HEALTH PRESS

Fast Facts: Multiple Myeloma and Plasma Cell Dyscrasias
First edition 2015
Second edition November 2017

Text © 2017 Karthik Ramasamy, Sagar Lonial
© 2017 in this edition Health Press Limited
Health Press Limited, Elizabeth House, Queen Street, Abingdon,
Oxford OX14 3LN, UK
Tel: +44 (0)1235 523233

Book orders can be placed by telephone or via the website.
For regional distributors or to order via the website, please go to:
www.fastfacts.com

For telephone orders, please call +44 (0)1752 202301.

Fast Facts is a trademark of Health Press Limited.

All rights reserved. No part of this publication may be reproduced, stored in a retrieval system, or transmitted in any form or by any means, electronic, mechanical, photocopying, recording or otherwise, without the express permission of the publisher.

The rights of Karthik Ramasamy and Sagar Lonial to be identified as the authors of this work have been asserted in accordance with the Copyright, Designs & Patents Act 1988 Sections 77 and 78.

The publisher and the authors have made every effort to ensure the accuracy of this book, but cannot accept responsibility for any errors or omissions.

For all drugs, please consult the product labeling approved in your country for prescribing information.

Registered names, trademarks, etc. used in this book, even when not marked as such, are not to be considered unprotected by law.

A CIP record for this title is available from the British Library.

ISBN 978-1-910797-33-4

Ramasamy K (Karthik)
Fast Facts: Multiple Myeloma and Plasma Cell Dyscrasias/
Karthik Ramasamy, Sagar Lonial

Medical illustrations by Annamaria Dutto, Withernsea, UK.
Typesetting by Thomas Bohm, User Design, Illustration and Typesetting, UK.
Printed in the UK with Xpedient Print.

List of abbreviations	4
Introduction	5
Epidemiology and etiology	7
Predisposing conditions associated with multiple myeloma	14
Pathophysiology of multiple myeloma and MGUS	28
Diagnosis, staging and monitoring of multiple myeloma	35
Genetics and multiple myeloma	51
Treatment of newly diagnosed multiple myeloma	57
Stem cell transplantation in multiple myeloma	71
Relapsed and refractory multiple myeloma	78
Bone disease and renal complications	98
AL amyloidosis	108
Rare plasma cell dyscrasias	122
Supportive care	137
Useful resources	150
Index	152

List of abbreviations

ADCC: antibody-dependent cell-mediated cytotoxicity

ADCP: antibody-dependent cellular phagocytosis

AIDS: autoimmune deficiency syndrome

AL amyloidosis: amyloid light-chain amyloidosis

allo-SCT: allogeneic stem cell transplantation

ASCT: autologous stem cell transplantation

ATTR: transthyretin amyloidosis

CDC: complement-dependent cytotoxicity

CKD: chronic kidney disease

CR: complete response

CRP: C-reactive protein

FDG: fludeoxyglucose

FISH: fluorescence in situ hybridization

FLC: free light chain

GEP: gene expression profiling

HDAC: histone deacetylase

HDT: high-dose therapy

HIV: human immunodeficiency virus

HLA: human leukocyte antigen

Ig: immunoglobulin

IMiD: immunomodulatory drug

IMWG: International Myeloma Working Group

ISS: International Staging System

LDH: lactate dehydrogenase

MGRS: monoclonal gammopathy of renal significance

MGSS: monoclonal gammopathy of skeletal significance

MGUS: monoclonal gammopathy of undetermined significance

MIDD: monoclonal immunoglobulin deposition disease

MM: multiple myeloma

MRI: magnetic resonance imaging

NT-proBNP: N-terminal pro-brain natriuretic peptide

OPG: osteoprogerin

PET-CT: positron emission tomography-computed tomography

POEMS: polyneuropathy, organomegaly, endocrinopathy, monoclonal gammopathy and skin changes (syndrome)

PR: partial response

RANKL: receptor activator of nuclear factor (NF)-κB ligand

RRMM: relapsed and refractory multiple myeloma

SAP: serum amyloid P

SCT: stem cell transplantation

sFLC: serum free light chain

VGPR: very good partial response

VTE: venous thromboembolism

WM: Waldenström's macroglobulinemia

Introduction

Our understanding of multiple myeloma (MM) is growing at a formidable pace, particularly in terms of risk factors and potential drug targets. Since the first edition of this *Fast Facts* handbook was published in 2015, the International Myeloma Working Group (IMWG) has published its new response criteria, which include minimal residual disease (MRD). Patients who achieve MRD negativity (< 0.01% abnormal plasma cells) have better outcomes than those with residual disease; thus, MRD negativity is set to become the new benchmark in clinical trials and treatment targets. The cytogenetic analysis of clonal plasma cells from patients with MRD is now also paving the way for personalized therapies, particularly for patients with high-risk disease, and the recently published revised International Staging System takes into account cytogenetic abnormalities in its risk stratification.

This second edition also includes the IMWG's recently extended definition of symptomatic MM to include histological and monoclonal protein criteria (the so-called SLiM CRAB criteria). The new criteria define a group of asymptomatic patients who have an extremely high risk of progression to symptomatic MM within 2 years and for whom delaying intervention could be detrimental. In light of this reclassification, 15% of patients with smoldering myeloma are eligible for standard MM treatment.

In Chapter 4 we describe the latest advances in diagnostic tests and imaging, while in Chapter 5 we discuss the current status of cytogenetics and genetic profiling; the identification of different subsets of MM heralds the advent of tailored treatment for individual patients based on cytogenetic risk factors.

Although MM remains incurable, our growing understanding of the disease and its premalignant stages is leading to better treatments. We have updated Chapters 6–8 to include recent advances in the treatment of MM. Induction therapy based on an immunomodulatory drug, a proteasome inhibitor and a steroid is now standard practice for patients eligible for stem cell transplantation (SCT), and lenalidomide-

and bortezomib-based regimens have replaced melphalan plus prednisone for patients who are not eligible for SCT. Although the myeloma community debates the necessity of SCT, clinical trials continue to show that high-dose therapy followed by autologous SCT provides significant benefits in terms of duration of remission and overall survival. Thus, it is incumbent on clinicians to treat to maximal response and to consider long-term therapeutic strategies – a third of patients can now expect to survive for 10 years or more from diagnosis.

Relapsed or refractory MM presents a different therapeutic challenge, requiring careful consideration of the balance between efficacy and toxicity in the choice of treatment: the emerging second-generation proteasome inhibitors, histone deacetylase inhibitors and the monoclonal antibodies provide a broader armamentarium for clinicians to work with.

This *Fast Facts* handbook provides a comprehensive overview of MM and other plasma cell dyscrasias, from bench to bedside, presenting the pathogenesis, diagnosis and treatment in the context of daily clinical practice. We believe it is an ideal resource for primary care providers, specialist nurses, junior doctors and allied healthcare professionals who want to get up to speed quickly in this fast-moving field.

You can quickly test your knowledge after reading this book by taking our FastTest at fastfacts.com, and please do post a comment for us on the site if you have any specific feedback. We hope that this book will help you to make better health decisions for all your patients with MM.

Acknowledgments. We thank Ms Charise Gleason, Department of Hematology and Medical Oncology, Winship Cancer Institute of Emory University, USA, for her coauthorship of Chapter 1. We also thank Drs Jaimal Kothari and Faye Sharpley from the Department of Clinical Haematology, Oxford University Hospitals NHS Trust, UK, for critical reading of the book, and Dr Debbie Hay for image contribution. We also thank Dr Dale Powner, Binding Site (UK), for providing images.

1 Epidemiology and etiology

Epidemiology

Multiple myeloma (MM) accounts for about 0.8% of all cancers worldwide, with about 114 000 new cases each year.[1] In the USA, it is the 14th most common cancer and the second most common hematologic malignancy. In Europe, it is the 20th most common cancer and the third most common hematologic malignancy.

Incidence and prevalence. The incidence of MM varies markedly across countries: the highest rates are reported in North America, parts of Europe, Australia and New Zealand, while the lowest rates are seen in Asia.

In the USA, the annual incidence of MM has increased by an average of 0.8% per year in the past decade, while death rates have been stable between 2002 and 2012. In 2012, an estimated 89 658 people were living with MM, and approximately 26 850 new cases were diagnosed in 2015. The estimated 5-year survival rate is 46.6%.

In Europe, up to 39 000 new cases of MM were diagnosed in 2012 (1% of total cancer cases), and the estimated age-standardized incidence was 4.5 per 100 000.[2] Cancer Research UK reported 4792 new cases of MM in 2011, with an age-standardized incidence of 5.4 per 100 000. In 2012, 24 000 myeloma-related deaths were reported, with an age-standardized mortality of 2.7 per 100 000 for men and 1.8 per 100 000 for women.[3] The 5-year prevalence of MM in Europe in 2012 was estimated at 89 191 cases.[4]

Etiology

The etiology of MM is not known, although a number of risk factors have been identified (Table 1.1).

Age. MM most commonly affects older adults. UK data show that the incidence of MM increases with age (Figure 1.1).[3] In the USA,

Fast Facts: Multiple Myeloma and Plasma Cell Dyscrasias

TABLE 1.1

Known risk factors for multiple myeloma

- Older age
- Male sex
- Personal history of MGUS
- Family history of multiple myeloma
- African or African American ethnicity

MGUS, monoclonal gammopathy of undetermined significance.

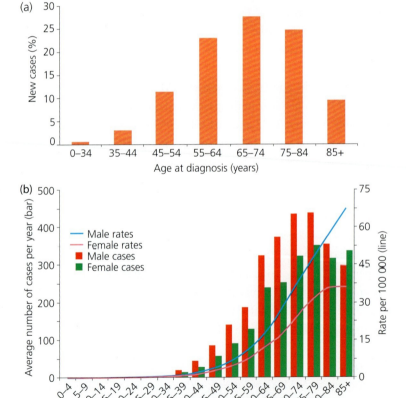

Figure 1.1 Incidence of multiple myeloma in relation to age in (a) the USA[5] and (b) the UK.[3]

Epidemiology and etiology

the median age at diagnosis is 69 years and fewer than 1% of cases are diagnosed before 35 years of age.

UK data for 2010–2012 also show that myeloma mortality rises with age. Mortality rates are highest in patients aged 75–84 years (Figure 1.2). Age-specific mortality rates of 55 (for men) and 33.1 (for women) per 100 000 have been reported in the over-85 year age group (see Figure 1.2). The median age at death in the USA is 75 years.

Sex. The incidence of MM is higher in men than in women across all ethnicities (Figure 1.3): rates of 7.9 versus 5.1 per 100 000 in men and

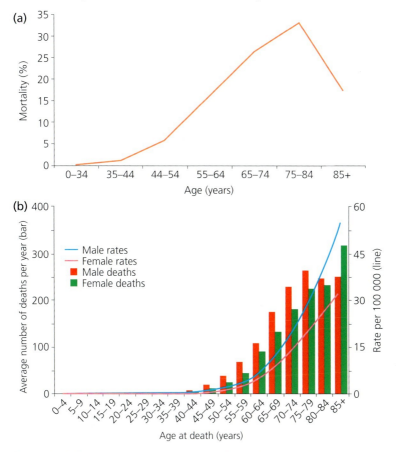

Figure 1.2 Mortality associated with multiple myeloma in relation to age in (a) the USA[5] and (b) the UK.[3]

women, respectively, in the USA,[5] and 4.7 versus 3.1 per 100 000 women in Europe[2] have been reported. Mortality rates in relation to sex reflect the differences in incidence, as shown in Figure 1.4.[5]

Ethnicity. African and African American populations are at higher risk of MM than are Caucasian populations; the risk is lowest in Asian populations (see Figure 1.3). Mortality rates in relation to ethnicity reflect the incidence, as shown in Figure 1.4, indicating that ethnicity does not markedly influence survival. However, new data suggest that the genetic presentation for MM is different in African Americans, with a higher incidence of hyperdiploid genetics and lower rates of $p53$ mutations. While African American patients may be 5–10 years

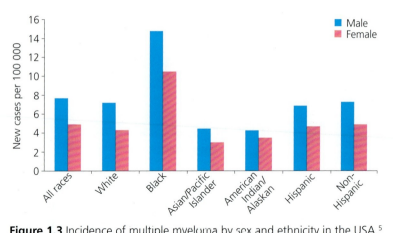

Figure 1.3 Incidence of multiple myeloma by sex and ethnicity in the USA.[5]

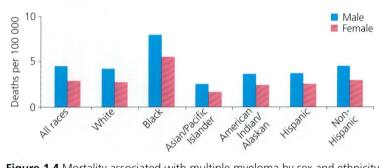

Figure 1.4 Mortality associated with multiple myeloma by sex and ethnicity in the USA.[5]

younger at presentation than patients of other ethnicities, their survival upon treatment with the new drugs is as good or better, attributed to the presence of fewer high-risk genetic changes. A recent genome-wide association study identified some key genetic loci that may explain the higher incidence of MM in African Americans compared with non-African Americans.

Family history and genetics. Several studies have shown that patients with a first-degree relative with MM or the precancerous condition monoclonal gammopathy of undetermined significance (MGUS; see Chapter 2) are more likely to develop MGUS or MM than those without a family history. To date, more than 100 families in whom several members have developed MM or other plasma cell dyscrasias have been described, providing strong evidence for an inherited component to the development of MM. The basis of this genetic contribution remains to be fully established, although studies have reported possible associations between myeloma risk and human leukocyte antigen (HLA) profiles, *BRCA1* and *BRCA2* mutations and single-nucleotide polymorphisms.[6–8]

Environmental factors. Several studies have explored the relationship between myeloma risk and environmental factors, including exposure to organic solvents, pesticides, hair dye and other chemicals, but results have been inconsistent. A possible association between MM and exposure to ionizing radiation has also been explored. A study of survivors of the atomic bomb in Japan reported that, in individuals exposed to 50 rad or more, an increased myeloma risk did not become apparent until at least 20 years after exposure. However, other studies suggest that exposure to radiation increases the incidence of MGUS (see Chapter 2) and also accelerates the transformation of MGUS to MM.

Obesity. Several studies have reported that obesity (body mass index ≥ 30 kg/m^2) is associated with an increased risk of MM or MGUS.[9,10]

Immunologic factors. Studies of the association between infections and the development of MM have yielded inconsistent results.[11] AIDS has been linked to an increased incidence of MGUS and MM, particularly in older patients; both HIV infection and immune dysfunction are associated with a higher prevalence of MGUS than in the general population but the role of HIV in the progression to MGUS or MM is not clear.

Key points – epidemiology and etiology

- Multiple myeloma (MM) accounts for about 0.8% of all cancers worldwide, with about 114 000 new cases each year.
- In the USA, it is the 14th most common cancer and the second most common hematologic malignancy. In Europe, it is the 20th most common cancer and the third most common hematologic malignancy.
- The incidence of MM is higher in men than in women, and increases with age – incidence is highest during the seventh decade.
- The risk of MM is highest in people of African or African American ethnicity and lowest in Asian populations. African American patients may be 5–10 years younger than white populations at presentation but their survival upon treatment with new drugs is as good or better, attributed to the presence of fewer high-risk genetic changes.
- There is evidence for a genetic risk for MM, although the basis for this remains to be established.
- There is no consistent evidence for an association between myeloma risk and any environmental factor.

References

1. World Cancer Research Fund International. *Cancer Facts and Figures: Worldwide Data*, 2015. www.wcrf.org/int/cancer-facts-figures/worldwide-data, last accessed 09 January 2017.

2. EUCAN http://eco.iarc.fr/eucan/Cancer.aspx?Cancer=39.

3. Cancer Research UK. *Myeloma Statistics 2015*. www.cancerresearch.org.uk/health-professional/cancer-statistics/statistics-by-cancer-type/myeloma, last accessed 09 January 2017.

4. Ferlay J, Steliarova-Foucher E, Lortet-Tieulent J et al. Cancer incidence and mortality patterns in Europe: estimates for 40 countries in 2012. *Eur J Cancer* 2013;49:1374–403.

5. National Cancer Institute. Surveillance, Epidemiology, and End Results Program. *SEER Stat Fact Sheets: Myeloma*, 2015. www.seer.cancer.gov/statfacts/html/mulmy.html, last accessed 09 January 2017.

6. Broderick P, Chubb D, Johnson DC et al. Common variation at 3p22.1 and 7p15.3 influences multiple myeloma risk. *Nat Genet* 2012;44:58–61.

7. Greenburg AJ, Rajkumar SV. Elucidating disparities across racial and ethnic groups in multiple myeloma patients. *Int J Hematol* 2012;95:453–4.

8. Morgan GJ, Johnson DC, Weinhold N et al. Inherited genetic susceptibility to multiple myeloma. *Leukemia* 2014;28:518–24.

9. Landgren O, Rajkumar V, Pfeiffer RM et al. Obesity is associated with an increased risk of monoclonal gammopathy of undetermined significance among black and white women. *Blood* 2010;116:1056–9.

10. Wallin A, Larsson SC. Body mass index and risk of multiple myeloma: a meta-analysis of prospective studies. *Eur J Cancer* 2011;47:1606–15.

11. Brown LM, Gridley G, Check D, Landgren O. Risk of multiple myeloma and monoclonal gammopathy of undetermined significance among white and black male United States veterans with prior autoimmune, infectious, and allergic disorders. *Blood* 2008;111:3388–94.

2 Predisposing conditions associated with multiple myeloma

Two predisposing conditions are associated with a risk of progression to multiple myeloma (MM):
- monoclonal gammopathy of undetermined significance (MGUS)
- asymptomatic or smoldering myeloma.

These differ in their clinical presentations, biochemical and cytological characteristics (Table 2.1) and risk of progression to MM.

MGUS

Definition. MGUS is a benign premalignant condition, defined as the presence of monoclonal immunoglobulin (Ig), referred to as M protein (also called paraprotein), in blood and/or urine but with no associated evidence of demonstrable end organ damage. The M protein is produced by plasma cells or lymphoplasmacytoid cells in the bone marrow. Patients with MGUS have elevated levels of immunoglobulin (Ig)G, IgA, IgM and/or serum free light chains in their blood.[1] The lifelong risk of progression to MM, lymphoma or amyloid light-chain (AL) amyloidosis (see Chapter 10) is 1% per annum.

Epidemiology. MGUS is one of the most common premalignant disorders in individuals over the age of 50 years.

Incidence. The incidence of MGUS increases with age but is difficult to determine accurately because data are limited. Population-wide registry studies from Iceland and the Netherlands have reported incidence rates of 9–31 per 100 000 person-years. Worldwide, the highest incidence of MGUS has been reported in survivors of the atomic bomb in Japan (164 per 100 000 person-years). Exposure to radiation is thought to increase the progression of MGUS to myeloma (see Chapter 1).

Prevalence rates of 0.3–6.2% have been reported, depending on the sensitivity of the tests used to measure M protein levels (see below) and the age, size and ethnicity of the population studied.

TABLE 2.1

Features of multiple myeloma and its precursors

	MGUS	Smoldering myeloma	MM
Symptoms	Asymptomatic	Asymptomatic	Symptomatic
M protein	Serum M protein < 3.0 g/dL or elevated serum FLC*	Serum M protein ≥ 3.0 g/dL and/or urinary M protein ≥ 500 mg/24 h	M protein in serum or urine
BM plasma cells	< 10%	10–59%	≥ 10% or biopsy-proven bony or extramedullary plasmacytoma
End organ damage	None	None	Evidence of end organ damage that can be attributed to the underlying lymphoproliferative disorder
Other	No other B cell proliferative disorder		• ≥ 1 biomarker of malignancy • clonal BM plasma cells ≥ 60% • involved:uninvolved serum FLC ratio ≥ 100, with iFLC > 100 mg/L • > 1 focal lesion on MRI studies

*See Table 2.2. BM, bone marrow; FLC, free light chain; iFLC, involved free light chain; MGUS, monoclonal gammopathy of undetermined significance; MM, multiple myeloma; MRI, magnetic resonance imaging.

The prevalence is up to fourfold higher in patients older than 80 years (6.6%) than in those aged 50–59 years, and the rate in men is double that in women.

The prevalence of MGUS is 2–3-fold higher among Africans or African Americans than in Caucasian populations but there is no difference between these ethnic groups in the rate of transformation to MM. The prevalence of MGUS is similar in African and African American populations, suggesting that the higher prevalence in these groups reflects a genetic predisposition rather than dietary or other environmental influences.

Etiology. Although the available evidence is inconsistent, occupational exposure to asbestos, aromatic hydrocarbons, fertilizers, mineral oils and petroleum, paints and related products, pesticides and radiation has been reported to be associated with an increased risk of MGUS.

Classification. The International Myeloma Working Group (IMWG) has defined three distinct clinical types of MGUS based on Ig profiles, as described in Table 2.2.

Diagnosis and evaluation. An isolated finding of serum M protein or elevated light chain levels should prompt further investigations to distinguish between MGUS and MM. The diagnosis of MGUS should only be made once tests confirm that there is no evidence of end organ damage secondary to the presence of M protein. End organ damage is assessed according to the CRAB criteria:
- Calcemia
- Renal insufficiency
- Anemia
- Bone lesions.

Blood tests, including a full blood count, renal profile and bone chemistry, should be carried out to identify any changes suggesting end organ damage.

Imaging should be performed to identify any myeloma-related bone changes, such as lytic lesions, vertebral compression fractures, significant osteopenia or osteoporosis. This often involves a radiographic skeletal survey, although other imaging techniques may also be helpful, as reviewed in Chapter 4 (see pages 41–42).

TABLE 2.2
Types of MGUS

	IgM	Non-IgM	Light-chain[1]
M protein	Presence of serum IgM (< 3.0 g/dL)	Presence of serum IgA or IgG (< 3.0 g/dL)	No heavy-chain Ig Abnormal FLC ratio (< 0.26 or > 1.65)*
BM involvement	Lymphoplasmacytic infiltration < 10%	Clonal BM plasma cells < 10%	Clonal BM plasma cells < 10%
End organ damage	None†	None‡	None‡
Potential to progress to (lifetime risk/ year)	Waldenström's macroglobulinemia, NHL or AL amyloidosis[6] (1.4%) IgM myeloma (very rare)	MM or a lymphoproliferative disorder (1%)	Light-chain myeloma (0.4%)

*Serum FLC ratio increases with declining renal function. Reference ratio of 0.26–3.1 applies here for patients with chronic kidney disease stages 3–5.
†No evidence of anemia, constitutional symptoms, hyperviscosity, lymphadenopathy, hepatosplenomegaly or other end organ damage that can be attributed to the underlying lymphoproliferative disorder.
‡Absence of end organ damage based on CRAB criteria ([hyper]Calcemia, Renal insufficiency, Anemia, Bone lesions) or amyloidosis that can be attributed to the plasma cell proliferative disorder.
AL, amyloid light-chain [amyloidosis]; BM, bone marrow; FLC, free light chain; Ig, immunoglobulin; MGUS, monoclonal gammopathy of undetermined significance; MGUS, monoclonal gammopathy of undetermined significance; MM, multiple myeloma; NHl, non-Hodgkin lymphoma.

End organ damage versus age-related organ dysfunction. It can be difficult to distinguish true end organ damage due to MM from age-related organ dysfunction from other causes. For example, age-related osteoporosis is common, requiring caution in diagnosing MGUS (or MM) on the basis of osteoporosis alone; lytic lesions or evidence of other organ damage is required for the diagnosis.

In addition to radiography, MRI or PET-CT may be helpful in difficult cases.

Similarly, chronic kidney disease is present in 30–50% of patients over 70 years of age, and is usually due to hypertension or diabetes; therefore, progression of MGUS to MM should not be diagnosed on the basis of renal dysfunction alone. Rarely, a renal biopsy may be required to determine whether monoclonal gammopathy is responsible for renal impairment.

If the degree of anemia seems disproportionately high compared with the level of M protein, MGUS or MM is unlikely to be the cause, and hematinic deficiency, chronic inflammation or even myelodysplastic syndrome should be considered. Finally, primary hyperparathyroidism, which is associated with mild hypercalcemia, is present in about 0.2% of patients over 70 years of age. Therefore, the presence of hypercalcemia should not trigger investigations to rule out conversion of MGUS to MM.

Risk profiling and progression. There are no specific genetic or phenotypic markers that distinguish MGUS from smoldering myeloma or MM. However, retrospective studies have identified several clinical parameters that are associated with an increased rate of progression from MGUS to MM (Table 2.3).

TABLE 2.3

Clinical parameters associated with increased risk of progression from MGUS to MM

- Increased monoclonal immunoglobulin (M protein) level
- Increased bone marrow plasmacytosis
- Abnormal free light chain ratio
- Non-immunoglobulin G isotype
- Immunoparesis (reduction in the levels of one or two uninvolved immunoglobulins)
- Abnormal plasma cells (aPC) > 95%
- Aneuploidy detected by flow cytometry

MGUS, monoclonal gammopathy of undetermined significance; MM, multiple myeloma.

Risk stratification models. Two models that predict the risk of progression from MGUS to myeloma have been developed, based on clinical markers. The most widely used model, developed by the Mayo Clinic, is based on three major risk factors:
- serum M protein > 1.5 g/dL (15 g/L)
- abnormal free light chain (FLC) ratio (< 0.26 or > 1.65)
- IgA, IgM or IgD (i.e. non-IgG isotype).

With this model, the absolute risk of progression to MM over 20 years is 5% for patients with none of these risk factors, increasing to 21%, 37% and 58% for patients with one, two or three, respectively (Table 2.4).

The risk model developed by scientists from Salamanca ('the Spanish group') uses two prognostic criteria based on the flow cytometry immunophenotypic profile of bone marrow plasma cells:[2]
- abnormal plasma cells (aPC) > 95%
- aneuploidy (abnormal chromosome numbers) characteristic of MGUS.

TABLE 2.4

Risk profiling schemes for the progression of MGUS to MM

No. of risk factors	No. of patients Mayo[5]/ Spanish[2]	Relative risk Mayo[5]/ Spanish[2]	Mayo[5] 20-year risk (%)*	Spanish[2] 5-year risk (%)
0	449 (39)/ 127 (46)	1.0/1.0	5/2	2
1	420 (37)/ 133 (48)	5.4/5.0	21/10	10
2	226 (20)/ 16 (6)	10.1/23.0	37/18	46
3	53 (5)/ –	20.8/ –	58/27	–

*Absolute risk/risk after accounting for competing causes of death.
Mayo clinic risk factors: M protein > 1.5 g/dL; non-immunoglobulin G monoclonal gammopathy of undetermined significance; free light chain ratio < 0.26 or > 1.65.[5]
Spanish group risk factors: ≥ 95% abnormal plasma cells; DNA aneuploidy.[2]
MGUS, monoclonal gammopathy of undetermined significance; MM, multiple myeloma.

With this model, patients with none of these risk factors have a risk of progression at 5 years of 2%, whereas this rises to 10% for those with one risk factor, and to 46% for those with two (see Table 2.4).

The Mayo model is simpler to use in clinical practice because it does not require a bone marrow test – recent guidance from the IMWG has stated that this is not required for patients with IgG MGUS and a normal serum FLC ratio. Risk profiling is routine practice now, but both methods are restricted to patients with conventional heavy-chain MGUS; neither is suitable for the more recently recognized light-chain MGUS.

Risk of progression to other plasma cell dyscrasias. In patients with IgM MGUS, the presence of both the L265P mutation in the *Myd88* gene and M protein levels above 1.5 g/dL is associated with a 45% risk of progression to Waldenström's macroglobulinemia, chronic lymphocytic leukemia or non-Hodgkin lymphoma over 10 years. Currently, there are no prognostic/risk profiling models that estimate the risk of progression from IgM MGUS to AL amyloidosis.

Long-term risks associated with MGUS are summarized in Table 2.5.

Poor life expectancy. Patients with MGUS have a compromised life expectancy compared with an age-adjusted normal population but this is not fully explained by the risk of progression to MM and other lymphoproliferative disorders.[3]

TABLE 2.5

Long-term risks of MGUS

- Reduced life expectancy
- Myeloid malignancies
- Infections
- Thrombosis
- Osteoporosis
- Heart disorders

MGUS, monoclonal gammopathy of undetermined significance.

Myeloid malignancies. Of most concern is the increased risk of myeloid malignancies in patients with MGUS, the only reasonable biological explanation for which is the changes in the bone marrow microenvironment. However, this could be a chance association, as patients with MGUS receive frequent surveillance; in addition, the prevalence of myeloid malignancies is increased in the elderly population, and those suspected of having malignancies are frequently given a serum electrophoresis test.

Thrombosis. Patients with MGUS have a 2–3-fold increased risk of thrombosis, particularly venous thrombosis, compared with the age-matched general population. The risk appears to be higher in patients with non-IgG MGUS with a higher M protein load. Higher levels of factor VIII and von Willebrand factor have been observed in these patients.

Infection. Studies have consistently shown that the risk of both bacterial and viral infections is increased up to twofold in patients with MGUS, who frequently have immunoparesis (reduced Ig levels) and low T-cell numbers.

Bone changes have also been well documented in patients with MGUS. The risk of osteoporosis is often increased in patients with MGUS, increasing the risk of fractures. For this reason, optimization of bone health should be considered for all patients with MGUS and appropriate investigations performed to exclude MM.

MGUS-associated disorders. Skeletal, renal, neuropathic and skin associations are increasingly being reported in patients with MGUS and there is a strong feeling among physicians that patients with MGUS should be subclassified into distinct groups based on these conditions, as set out below.

Monoclonal gammopathy of renal significance (MGRS). Renal damage can result from deposition of both light and heavy chains in the glomeruli and renal tubules. The generic term MGRS covers a number of abnormalities seen in renal biopsies:
- crystallization
- cryoglobulin formation
- amyloid formation
- glomerulonephritis induced by M protein.

Ways to identify at-risk patients are needed, followed by clinical trials to determine whether early therapy can prevent irreversible renal damage.

Monoclonal gammopathy of skeletal significance (MGSS). As noted above, the risk of fractures is increased in patients with MGUS, and the prevalence of MGUS is higher in patients with osteoporosis, which is thought to be due to osteoclast activation and osteoblast suppression (as seen in MM). However, in clinical studies, markers of bone turnover and dual-energy X-ray absorptiometry have not predicted increased fracture risk in patients with MGUS. Improvement of bone health through general lifestyle measures, such as smoking cessation, weight optimization and adequate calcium and vitamin D intake, may modify this risk.

MGUS-associated neuropathy. IgM MGUS is frequently associated with neuropathy, and patients often have antibodies against myelin-associated glycoprotein and other neural proteins. Patients with non-IgM MGUS also present with neuropathy, although the pathogenesis for this remains unclear; underlying lymphoproliferative disorders must be excluded.

Neuropathy is a predominant feature in patients with POEMS syndrome (polyneuropathy, organomegaly, endocrinopathy, monoclonal gammopathy and skin changes) and AL amyloidosis, and often presents when there are low levels of M protein. The presentation and management of these conditions is discussed in Chapters 10 and 11.

MGUS-associated dermopathy. Type 1 cryoglobulinemia (monoclonal) is associated with the presence of M protein and skin lesions (Figure 2.1), and treatment of this underlying gammopathy is likely to improve skin manifestations. Schnitzler syndrome presents as an urticarial-type skin rash, arthralgia, bone pain, lymphadenopathy and abnormal IgM. Treatment with anakinra (an interleukin-1 receptor antagonist) induces significant responses in these patients. Scleromyxedema, scleredema, xanthoma and necrobiotic xanthogranuloma are other rare skin conditions associated with MGUS.

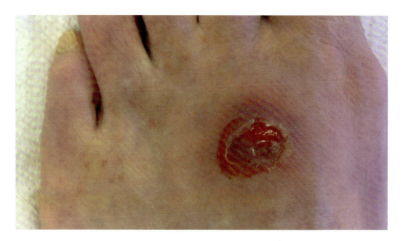

Figure 2.1 Dermopathy associated with monoclonal gammopathy of undetermined significance – skin lesion on the foot.

Monitoring and referral. If tested, a large proportion of patients over the age of 50 years would be found to have MGUS. The algorithm shown in Figure 2.2 has been developed to guide the monitoring of these patients and indicates when referral to secondary care is required. In principle, patients with a low to intermediate risk of progression require infrequent monitoring in the community. However, high-risk patients should be reviewed in secondary care and followed up or discharged to primary care with clear instructions for re-referral, as should patients in whom it is unclear whether the M protein is the cause of other subtle changes in organ function.

Smoldering myeloma

Epidemiology. Smoldering myeloma is a malignant condition and accounts for about 14% of all newly diagnosed cases of myeloma.

Definition. Traditionally, smoldering myeloma has been defined by the presence of more than 10% plasma cells in the bone marrow or an M protein level above 3.0 g/dL, but without any of the clinical end organ damage (CRAB criteria; see page 16) that conventionally defines symptomatic MM.

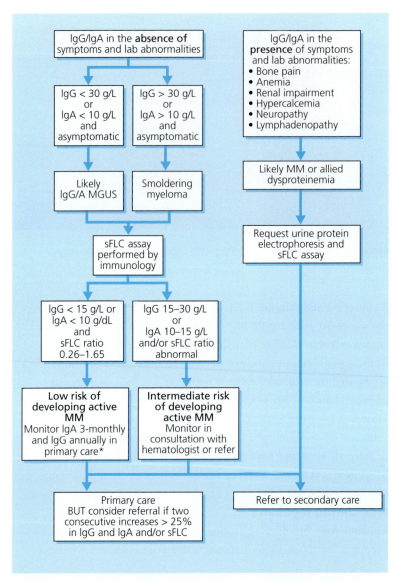

Figure 2.2 Use of immunoglobulin (Ig) levels and serum free light chain (sFLC) ratio to guide monitoring of patients with MGUS in primary care, and referral to secondary care. *Full blood count, renal and bone profile, sFLC assay, serum electrophoresis and paraprotein measurement. MGUS, monoclonal gammopathy of undetermined significance; MM, multiple myeloma.

Risk of progression. Smoldering myeloma has a risk of progression to symptomatic disease of about 10% per year for the first 5 years, after which the risk diminishes. In about 25% of patients, smoldering myeloma behaves biologically as stable MGUS, and does not progress to symptomatic disease. Smoldering myeloma therefore includes a biological spectrum ranging from non-progressive premalignant MGUS to tumors that inevitably progress to symptomatic disease.[4]

Although efforts have been made to identify biomarkers that predict the risk of progression from MGUS or smoldering myeloma to symptomatic disease, there has been a lack of concordance and validation of biomarkers for smoldering myeloma. The IMWG published a revised definition of MM in 2014, which incorporated three new criteria in addition to the established CRAB criteria for initiating therapy (see page 16). These 'SliM CRAB' criteria are based on:

- Sixty percent ($\geq 60\%$) aPCs in the bone marrow
- Light chain levels – serum FLC (sFLC) ratio greater than 100[5]
- MRI findings – the presence of more than one focal lesion on advanced imaging (low-dose whole-body CT, MRI or ^{18}FDG-PET).

These new criteria define a group of otherwise asymptomatic patients who have an extremely high risk of progression to symptomatic MM within 2 years and for whom delaying intervention could be detrimental. In light of this reclassification, 15% of patients with smoldering myeloma are eligible for standard MM treatment. Studies are under way to establish whether earlier treatment of high-risk smoldering myeloma can delay end organ damage, improve survival and achieve cure.

A number of factors influence the risk of progression to MM in the remaining patients with smoldering myeloma. Table 2.6 summarizes risk factors reported by the Mayo Clinic and Danish and Spanish myeloma research groups. Patients with the highest risk of progression to myeloma are recruited into clinical trials.

TABLE 2.6

Risk factors for progression from smoldering myeloma to multiple myeloma, based on three risk models

No. risk factors	Mayo Clinic* (n = 273)			Spanish group† (n = 106)		Danish group‡ (n = 297)		
	Risk of progression		% of total	Risk of progression at 5 years	% of total	Risk of progression		% of total
	5 yrs	10 yrs				2 yrs	5 yrs	
0	–	–	–	4	36.8	4.8	9	30.3
1	25	50	29.7	46	36.8	18.1	24	55.6
2	51	65	41.8	72	26.4	38.4	55	14.1
3	76	84	28.6	–	–	–	–	–

Values are % risk of progression.
*Bone marrow plasma cells ≥ 10%, M protein ≥ 30 g/dL, free light chain ratio < 0.125 or > 8.[7]
†≥ 95% aberrant bone marrow plasma cells; immunoparesis (reduction in the levels of one or two uninvolved immunoglobulins).[2]
‡M protein ≥ 30 g/dL; immunoparesis.[8]
Adapted from Van de Donk, 2016.[9]

Key points – predisposing conditions associated with multiple myeloma

- The incidence of monoclonal gammopathy of undetermined significance (MGUS) increases with age: the condition is present in 5–8% of those over 70 years of age in the western world. Overall survival of these older patients is shorter than that of the age-adjusted non-MGUS population.
- Immunoglobulin (Ig)G or A MGUS progresses to myeloma or a lymphoproliferative disorder; IgM MGUS progresses to Waldenström's macroglobulinemia, non-Hodgkin lymphoma or amyloid light-chain amyloidosis. Light-chain MGUS progresses to light-chain myeloma.
- Risk profiling of patients with MGUS can help to identify those at high risk of progression.

(CONTINUED)

> **Key points** (CONTINUED)
>
> - Cutaneous, neurological, renal and skeletal manifestations have increasingly been noted in patients with MGUS.
> - Risk factors for high risk of progression from smoldering myeloma to MM within 2 years have been defined; these patients are now eligible for therapy in the new classification.

References

1. Dispenzieri A, Katzmann JA, Kyle RA et al. Prevalence and risk of progression of light-chain monoclonal gammopathy of undetermined significance: a retrospective population-based cohort study. *Lancet* 2010;375:1721–8.

2. Pérez-Persona E, Vidriales MB, Mateo G et al. New criteria to identify risk of progression in monoclonal gammopathy of uncertain significance and smoldering multiple myeloma based on multiparameter flow cytometry analysis of bone marrow plasma cells. *Blood* 2007;110:2586–92.

3. Kristinsson SY, Björkholm M, Andersson TM et al. Patterns of survival and causes of death following a diagnosis of monoclonal gammopathy of undetermined significance: a population-based study. *Haematologica* 2009;94:1714–20.

4. Rajkumar SV, Landgren O, Mateos M-V. Smoldering multiple myeloma. *Blood* 2015;125:3069–75.

5. Rajkumar SV, Kyle RA, Therneau TM et al. Serum free light chain ratio is an independent risk factor for progression in monoclonal gammopathy of undetermined significance. *Blood* 2005;106:812–17.

6. Kyle RA, Therneau TM, Rajkumar SV et al. Long-term follow-up of IgM monoclonal gammopathy of undetermined significance. *Blood* 2003;102:3759–64.

7. Dispenzieri A, Kyle RA, Katzmann JA et al. Immunoglobulin free light chain ratio is an independent risk factor for progression of smoldering (asymptomatic) multiple myeloma. *Blood* 2008;111:785–9.

8. Sørrig R, Klausen TW, Salomo M et al. Smoldering multiple myeloma risk factors for progression: a Danish population-based cohort study. *Eur J Haematol* 2016;97:303–9.

9. van de Donk NW, Mutis T, Poddighe PJ et al. Diagnosis, risk stratification and management of monoclonal gammopathy of undetermined significance and smoldering multiple myeloma. *Int J Lab Hematol* 2016;38(Suppl 1):110–22.

3   Pathophysiology of multiple myeloma and MGUS

Multiple myeloma (MM) is a disorder of clonal plasma cells – immune effector cells derived from bone marrow B cells following activation by antigens. The malignant plasma cells secrete abnormal antibodies, which accumulate in the body, resulting in hematologic, renal and skeletal complications. The signs of active myeloma and the associated organ damage relate at least partly to interactions between the malignant plasma cells and other cells within the bone marrow: these interactions fuel survival of the plasma cell clone and probably contribute to the development of induced drug resistance.

Studies have shown that patients with myeloma almost universally have a premalignant stage: monoclonal gammopathy of undetermined significance (MGUS; see Chapter 2).

Normal plasma cell development

During early B-cell differentiation in the bone marrow, the variable (V), diversity (D) and joining (J) segments of the immunoglobulin (Ig) genes are randomly assembled (somatic VDJ recombination) to generate unique receptors that can recognize different antigens. This process generates the antibody diversity needed for a healthy immune system. B cells have a protein complex on the cell surface, called the B cell receptor, that allows the B cell to escape apoptosis and proceed from the bone marrow to the lymph nodes (Figure 3.1). Here, undifferentiated precursor B cells from the bone marrow are transformed into mature B cells, which respond to a limited number of antigens. This primary immune response generates pre-germinal-center B cells, which are generally short-lived and usually secrete immunoglobulin (Ig)M. However, some of the antigen-activated cells enter the germinal center of the lymph nodes where they undergo clonal proliferation (Figure 3.2). The resulting clonal plasma cells undergo several rounds of somatic hypermutation, which introduces

Pathophysiology of multiple myeloma and MGUS

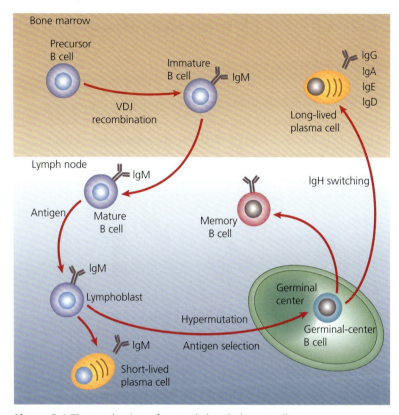

Figure 3.1 The production of normal clonal plasma cells.

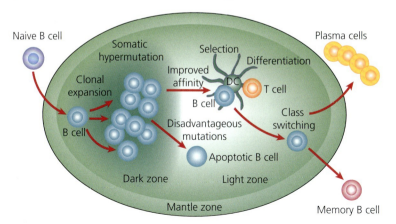

Figure 3.2 Clonal proliferation of B cells in the germinal center of a lymph node, and differentiation into plasma B cells (see text). DC, dendritic cell.

mutations into regions of the Ig genes, refining the antigen specificity of the Ig molecule.

Each clonal plasma cell synthesizes one specific Ig, consisting of two identical heavy chains and two identical light chains (Figure 3.3). These cells subsequently differentiate into memory B cells or post-germinal-center plasmablasts/plasma cells, either of which may undergo Ig heavy chain (IgH) switch recombination; this switches

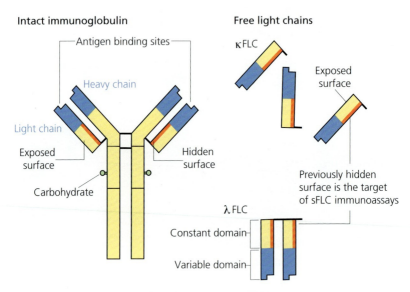

Figure 3.3 Every immunoglobulin (Ig) molecule comprises two identical heavy chains and two identical light chains. Each heavy chain is paired with a light chain, of which there are two serologically distinguishable types: kappa (κ) and lambda (λ). Ig molecules in plasma cells have either κ or λ light chain types, but never both. B cells produce either κ or λ light chains, which associate with heavy chains; however, more light chains than heavy chains are produced; those that remain unbound are secreted into the blood as free light chains (FLCs). In healthy individuals, the ratio of circulating κ and λ FLCs ranges from 0.26 to 1.65. Several conditions, such as kidney disease or inflammatory disorders, can cause elevations in serum FLCs (sFLC) but in these cases *both* κ and λ are affected equally and hence the ratio remains within the normal range. An abnormal ratio indicates a monoclonal gammopathy.

the class of Ig expressed by the cell – usually to IgG or IgA – after which the cells typically migrate back to the bone marrow, where they become terminally differentiated long-lived plasma cells (see Figure 3.1).

MGUS

In MGUS, the process of isotype switching becomes disordered. The resultant aberrant clonal plasma cells retain many of the phenotypic properties of healthy cells but proliferate slowly. Furthermore, studies have not shown any significant differences between the phenotypes of plasma cells found in MGUS and those of MM, and there are no significant differences in the gene expression profiles of the plasma cells. Although there may be additional epigenetic changes (i.e. changes that occur in a chromosome without affecting the DNA sequence) and differences in microRNA expression between MGUS and MM, these changes are not thought to be responsible for progression from MGUS to MM. Rather, the transition is thought to be due to expansion of the MGUS clonal cell population over time.

Transition to myeloma

MM is characterized by a change in plasma cells, resulting in the formation of a clonal population of tumor cells that no longer express surface antigen receptors but secrete large amounts of antibodies (referred to as M protein or paraprotein), or Ig light chains that accumulate in the serum, urine or both. This change in plasma cells is mediated by down-regulation of the *Pax5* gene and up-regulation of the transcription factors BLIMP1, IRF4 and XBP1s.

A number of genetic abnormalities that may influence the transformation of normal plasma cells into precancerous or myeloma cells have been reported in both MM and MGUS (Table 3.1). In general, patients who present with MGUS or symptomatic myeloma have similar genetic charactcristics, although there is evidence that certain genetic mutations, notably increased *MYC* expression or *KRAS* mutations, may influence the transition from MGUS to myeloma.[1]

TABLE 3.1
Genetic abnormalities observed in multiple myeloma

Event	Examples
Ig translocations (cyclin D family)	11q13, 6p21, 12p13
Ig translocations (MAF 2 family)	16q23, 20q12, 8q24
Ig translocations (MMSET/FGFR3)	4p16
Hyperdiploid (trisomy)	3, 5, 7, 9, 11, 15, 19, 21
Chromosome deletions	13p, 17p, 1p, 6q
Chromosome gains	1q

Ig, immunoglobulin.

The importance of the bone marrow microenvironment

Myeloma plasma cells typically co-exist with normal plasma cells in the bone marrow microenvironment, and the two cell types depend on the same survival cues in this environment, including locally produced soluble cytokines and direct cell interactions.[2] The survival of both long-lived plasma cells and myeloma cells is maintained by expression of induced myeloid leukemia cell differentiation protein Mcl-1. The survival of myeloma cells in the bone marrow microenvironment also requires a number of cytokines and trophic factors (Table 3.2). In particular, interleukin-6, which is secreted by both plasma cells and stromal cells within the bone marrow, is an important cytokine in the

TABLE 3.2
Cytokines implicated in maintaining a favorable microenvironment for myeloma cells in the bone marrow

- Interleukin (IL)-6
- Tumor necrosis factor (TNF)
- Vascular endothelial growth factor (VEGF)
- Dickkopf-related protein 1 (DKK1)
- B cell-activating factor (BAFF)

bone marrow microenvironment because it activates the Ras/Raf/MAPK pathway, which leads to survival and proliferation of the malignant clone.[3] Similarly, tumor necrosis factor plays an important role in stimulating proliferation of the malignant clone and inducing drug resistance in tumor cells.

The importance of the plasma cell microenvironment for survival and proliferation of the malignant clone is highlighted by the growing focus on cytokines and growth factors in the bone marrow as therapeutic targets.

Biological basis for current treatments

The introduction of proteasome inhibitors such as bortezomib has had an important impact on the survival of patients with myeloma. Proteasomes are cellular complexes that break down tumor suppressor proteins such as p53. The rationale for inhibition of the proteasome as a therapeutic approach was initially based on inhibition of the nuclear factor (NF)-κB signaling pathway, but there is also evidence that proteasomes are important in maintaining the quality of the large amounts of Ig proteins produced by plasma cells. Thus, an agent that interferes with normal protein homeostasis in the context of large-scale protein production may attack the 'Achilles heel' of plasma cells. Newer products in this class include the reversible inhibitor ixazomib and the irreversible inhibitor carfilzomib, which are better tolerated than bortezomib (a reversible inhibitor), enabling continuous administration. These are described in more detail in Chapter 6.

Myeloma cells may also display significant genomic instability and may therefore be more dependent than normal cells on DNA repair processes. This may at least partly explain why myeloma cells are sensitive to alkylating agents such as cyclophosphamide, bendamustine or melphalan. Furthermore, inhibition of DNA repair may contribute to the activity of proteasome inhibitors, creating a potential rationale for the combination of proteasome inhibitors with alkylating agents.

An alternative approach to the treatment of myeloma has been to use immunomodulatory drugs such as the combination of thalidomide with dexamethasone. Although these agents were previously believed to act by inhibiting angiogenesis, accumulating evidence suggests that they inhibit proteasome function by binding to a protein known as cereblon, resulting in an antiproliferative effect on myeloma cells.

> **Key points – pathophysiology of multiple myeloma and MGUS**
>
> - Multiple myeloma invariably has a premalignant stage (monoclonal gammopathy of undetermined significance; MGUS) of variable duration.
> - No significant differences between the phenotype and genotype profiles of myeloma and MGUS plasma cells have been identified.
> - Survival of myeloma cells in the bone marrow is dependent on a permissive microenvironment.
> - Cytokines drive proliferation of plasma cells and enhance survival.

References

1. Kuehl WM, Bergsagel PL. Molecular pathogenesis of multiple myeloma and its premalignant precursor. *J Clin Invest* 2012;122:3456–63.

2. Bianchi G, Anderson KC. Understanding biology to tackle the disease: multiple myeloma from bench to bedside, and back. *CA Cancer J Clin* 2014;64:422–44.

3. Moser K, Tokoyoda K, Radbruch A et al. Stromal niches, plasma cell differentiation and survival. *Curr Opin Immunol* 2006;18:265–70.

4 Diagnosis, staging and monitoring of multiple myeloma

Multiple myeloma (MM) is a heterogeneous disorder which, as described in Chapters 2 and 3, is invariably preceded by a premalignant stage. Early diagnosis is critical for a favorable outcome, but diagnosis is often delayed. In the UK, for example, a patient will typically have three appointments with a primary care practitioner over 6 months or longer before myeloma is suspected. However, the 6 months from the development of symptoms to diagnosis is critical, because delay often results in life-threatening comorbidities such as renal impairment requiring dialysis or fracture leading to spinal cord compression.

Early diagnosis is crucial to improve clinical outcomes

Signs and symptoms

Patients with MM often present with fatigue, bone pain or fractures, infections and renal impairment. Unexplained anemia, renal impairment, fatigue, fracture, osteoporosis and recurrent infections should alert the physician to a likely diagnosis of MM.

A comprehensive medical history should be taken, focusing on comorbid conditions that may affect treatment decisions, such as ischemic heart disease, heart failure, hypertension, renal disorders, liver disorders, neuropathy and lung pathology. A formal assessment of performance status (general well-being and activities of daily living) is also important.

Blood and urine tests

Initial investigation of a patient with suspected myeloma should include blood and urine tests (Table 4.1).[1]

TABLE 4.1
Diagnostic tests for multiple myeloma
- Complete and differential blood count; peripheral blood smear
- Bone, liver and renal biochemistry profile, including:
  – albumin
  – calcium
  – creatinine
  – lactate dehydrogenase
- Serum β_2-microglobulin
- Quantification of serum immunoglobulins
- Serum electrophoresis, immunofixation
- Routine urinalysis, 24-hour urine collection for electrophoresis and immunofixation
- Measurement of serum free light chains
- Spine and pelvis MRI
- Bone marrow aspirate and trephine biopsy
- Fluorescence in situ hybridization (FISH) on purified bone marrow cells
- Radiographic skeletal bone survey, including spine, ribs, pelvis, skull, humeri and femurs

Complete blood count and peripheral blood smear. Complete and differential blood counts should be ordered, and a peripheral blood smear evaluated for Rouleaux formations (stacking or aggregation of red blood cells; Figure 4.1) and circulating plasma cells.

Anemia is a common presenting feature of myeloma. However, if the degree of anemia is disproportionate to the tumor load (i.e. based on the level of M protein and number of plasma cells in the bone marrow), other causes should be ruled out, such as iron or vitamin deficiencies. Lymphopenia is a common finding, and neutropenia may also be observed in some cases. Red cell macrocytosis is often also noted, although this may be an artifact resulting from the presence of paraprotein.

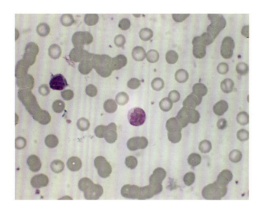

Figure 4.1 Blood film from a patient with multiple myeloma, showing Rouleaux formations (stacking of red blood cells) and mature plasma cells.

Bone, liver and renal biochemistry. A complete biochemistry panel, including liver function tests, renal profile and bone profile, is required. Renal function is abnormal in up to one-third of patients with newly diagnosed myeloma, and early treatment can restore renal function in most cases. Raised alkaline phosphatase may be observed in patients with recent fractures, and occasionally in patients with coexisting amyloid light-chain (AL) amyloidosis. High lactate dehydrogenase (LDH) levels indicate tumor proliferation and poor prognosis. Low serum albumin also indicates a poor prognosis.

Hypercalcemia is common at diagnosis, because osteolysis, which predominates in patients with myeloma, causes calcium to leach out of the bone. Patients often develop symptomatic hypercalcemia, requiring treatment with bisphosphonates. If mild or moderate hypercalcemia is detected in the absence of typical myeloma bone lesions, the possibility of primary hyperparathyroidism should be ruled out by measurement of serum parathyroid hormone level and referral to an endocrinologist.

Serum protein electrophoresis and immunofixation. Levels of serum immunoglobulins (Ig) should be measured in all patients, and serum immunofixation performed. Patients with MM commonly have immunoparesis – a decrease in Ig value to below normal levels. Serum immunofixation is required to confirm the presence of M protein and to subtype the clonal (Ig) protein (Figure 4.2).

Serum immunofixation should also be performed if myeloma or a related disorder is suspected and there is hypogammaglobulinemia or

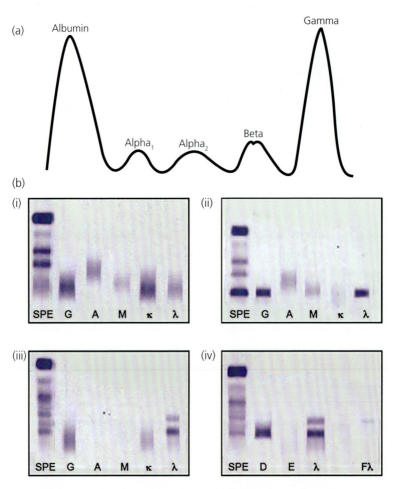

Figure 4.2 The presence of monoclonal (M) protein in myeloma is confirmed by an abnormal serum protein electrophoresis (SPE) pattern. (a) Typically, a homogeneous spike in a focal region of the gamma globulin zone is seen in monoclonal gammopathies. (b) SPE and immunofixation panels: (i) immunoglobulin (Ig)Gκ (ii) IgGλ (iii) λ light chain; (iv) IgDλ. Reproduced courtesy of Me Musset, Hôpital Pitié-Salpétrière, Paris, France.

the serum electrophoretic pattern appears normal. When a patient has only monoclonal light chains or serum M protein but immunofixation is negative for IgG, IgA or IgM, the possibility of IgD or IgE monoclonal paraproteinemia must be considered.

Urine protein electrophoresis and immunofixation should be performed in parallel with serum assays, and a 24-hour urine collection obtained to calculate the degree of proteinuria. An aliquot from an adequately concentrated 24-hour specimen should be sent for electrophoresis and immunofixation.

Measurement of serum free light chains (sFLCs) is recommended in all patients with newly diagnosed plasma cell dyscrasias, and an sFLC assay (see Figure 3.3, page 30) is now widely available. Measurement of sFLC is particularly useful in patients with oligosecretory myeloma, in which small amounts of M protein are secreted in the serum, urine or both. An sFLC assay is also useful for the diagnosis and monitoring of light-chain myeloma.

In patients with renal impairment, the half-life, and thus the serum concentration, of sFLC can increase tenfold, resulting in an abnormal $\kappa:\lambda$ ratio (see Figure 3.3), which can be used for diagnosis and monitoring. Recent studies have shown that measurement of sFLC also provides a sensitive assessment of response to treatment in patients with myeloma.

Measurement of β_2-microglobulin, a marker of tumor load, should be included in initial testing. The International Staging System (ISS) for MM uses both β_2-microglobulin and serum albumin levels to determine prognosis in patients with MM (Table 4.2). Patients with renal impairment due to MM have markedly elevated β_2-microglobulin levels.

Renal biopsy
Some patients with myeloma and comorbid diabetes or hypertension may have non-selective proteinuria associated with mild to moderate but stable renal impairment. A renal biopsy may be indicated in this situation to rule out renal lesions related to a plasma cell disorder, because such lesions usually progress to end-stage renal disease.

Bone marrow examination
Unilateral bone marrow aspiration alone may be sufficient to confirm the diagnosis but trephine biopsy allows better assessment of the

TABLE 4.2
International Staging System for multiple myeloma*

Stage	Serum β_2-microglobulin (mg/L)	Serum albumin (g/dL)	Median survival (months)†
I	< 3.5	≥ 3.5	62
II (i.e., not I or III)	3.5–5.5	Any	44
	< 3.5	< 3.5	
III	≥ 5.5		29

*See page 42.
†Historical survival data, when the International Staging System was defined. Survival is improving with newer treatments.

extent of marrow infiltration than aspirate smears. An adequate trephine biopsy (≥ 20 mm in length) should be obtained at the same time as the bone marrow aspiration, in order to avoid a repeat procedure if the aspirate proves inadequate.

Plasma cell phenotyping to distinguish between normal and neoplastic plasma cells may be performed by flow cytometry, immunohistochemistry or both. The European Myeloma Network has provided practical guidance on optimal flow cytometry procedures, and rapid and cost-effective single-tube assays have been developed.

The percentage of plasma cells in the bone marrow is currently determined on the basis of morphological assessment rather than flow cytometry. CD138 immunostaining of trephine sections can be useful to determine the extent of infiltration in selected cases.

The clonality of plasma cells should be established using immunoperoxidase staining. Some centers use flow cytometry to perform immunophenotyping but this is not widely available.

The presence of more than 10% clonal plasma cells on morphological examination of stained bone marrow aspirates and trephine sections confirms the diagnosis of MM (Figure 4.3). When both procedures are performed, the higher number of plasma cells obtained is used for diagnosis. The diagnosis of MM requires

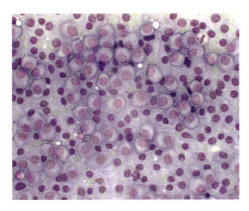

Figure 4.3 Bone marrow aspirate from a patient with multiple myeloma, showing numerous plasma cells with characteristic eccentric nucleus and perinuclear halo.

demonstration of abnormal plasma cells, monoclonality (i.e. secreting a single type of antibody) or both.

Imaging

Skeletal radiography is widely used to identify areas of bone damage in patients with MM (Figure 4.4) and is the screening technique of choice at diagnosis, although it has low sensitivity. Low-dose whole-body CT is therefore increasingly being used as a screening tool. The skeletal survey should include a postero-anterior view of the chest, anteroposterior (AP) and lateral views of the cervical spine, thoracic spine, lumbar spine, humeri and femora, AP and lateral views of the skull, and an AP view of the pelvis; other symptomatic painful areas

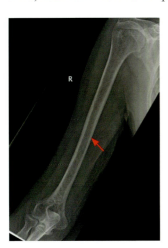

Figure 4.4 Skeletal radiography reveals lytic lesions in long bones and the skull. Here, lytic lesions can be seen in the humerus. See also Figure 9.1, page 99.

should be specifically visualized with appropriate views or advanced imaging techniques (see below).

CT and MRI provide higher sensitivity than skeletal radiography in the identification of bone lesions and are becoming more important in the determination of prognosis. CT or MRI of specific bone sites is useful for characterizing the bone changes seen on skeletal radiography. These results are often required in multidisciplinary team meetings to inform decisions about use of surgery or radiotherapy in addition to systemic therapy to ameliorate bone lesions. CT and MRI are the only modalities that can provide useful information about soft tissue plasmacytomas (tumors) and, occasionally, extramedullary disease.

Bone scintigraphy has no place in the routine staging of MM, and sequential dual-energy X-ray absorptiometry is not recommended, although it may detect early osteopenia or osteoporosis in patients with smoldering myeloma who might benefit from bisphosphonate therapy. PET-CT and 2-methoxyisobutylisonitrile (MIBI) imaging are also not recommended for routine use in the management of myeloma patients. Clinical trials are investigating the role of PET-CT and other radionuclide scans in diagnosis, determining prognosis and assessing response in patients with MM.

Staging and risk stratification

The survival of patients with myeloma varies from a few months to a few decades, even with several new classes of treatment. A staging system is therefore needed to determine the extent of tumor burden and hence the likely prognosis.

Staging. The Durie and Salmon staging system, published in 1975, determined tumor burden on the basis of blood counts, size of clonal protein, renal and bone biochemistry and skeletal imaging. However, this was superseded in 2005 by the ISS, which defines three risk categories on the basis of serum concentration of β_2-microglobulin and albumin (see Table 4.2). The ISS applies to patients who are symptomatic according to the CRAB criteria (see page 16); therefore, patients with ISS stage I MM are not considered to have smoldering myeloma. Patients with ISS stage III MM are considered to be at high risk of adverse outcomes. The ISS remains prognostic despite improvements in survival through advances in anti-myeloma therapy.[2]

Several cytogenetic and molecular genetic abnormalities have been identified that could provide useful prognostic information, listed in Table 4.3. These markers are associated with adverse outcomes, and it has been proposed that these abnormalities define high-risk myeloma and should therefore be specifically sought at diagnosis in all patients. The recently published revised ISS (rISS) combines some of the fundamentals of the ISS (β_2-microglobulin and albumin) with features known to be associated with poor outcomes, such as elevated LDH and the presence of del(17p), t(4;14), t(14;16) and t(14;20) chromosomal alterations, as shown in Table 4.4.[3] The rISS has become the standard method for defining populations and reporting in trials.

Risk stratification has been attempted in order to define specific pathways of clinical management. Studies in the USA and EU have shown that gene expression profiling (GEP) can be individually prognostic but there was minimal overlap in the genes identified in these studies, reflecting the different methods used to generate the GEP signature and variation in the underlying biology in high-risk myeloma. Some of the GEP signatures have been validated as independent prognostic factors, and the prognostic utility of others

TABLE 4.3

Genetic markers associated with adverse outcomes

- Immunoglobulin heavy chain gene translocations:
  - t(4;14)
  - t(14;16)
  - t(14;20)
- Copy number changes:
  - 1q gain
  - 1p loss
  - 17p deletion

TABLE 4.4

Standard risk factors for multiple myeloma and the rISS[2]

	Prognostic factor	Criteria
ISS stage	I	Serum β_2-microglobulin < 3.5 mg/L
		Serum albumin ≥ 3.5 g/dL
	II	Not ISS stage I or III
	III	Serum β_2-microglobulin ≥ 5.5 mg/L
CA by iFISH	High risk	Presence of at least one of: • del(17p) • translocation t(4;14), t(4;16) or t(4;20)
	Standard risk	No high-risk abnormalities
LDH	Normal	Serum LDH < ULN
	High	Serum LDH > ULN
A new model for risk stratification for MM	I	ISS stage I and standard-risk CA by iFISH and normal LDH
	II	Not rISS stage I or III
	III	ISS stage III and either high-risk CA by iFISH or high LDH

CA, chromosomal abnormalities; iFISH, interphase fluorescent in situ hybridization; ISS, International Staging System; LDH, lactate dehydrogenase; MM, multiple myeloma; rISS, revised International Staging System.

is being evaluated prospectively in clinical trials. The rISS developed by the International Myeloma Working Group (IMWG) provides a risk stratification on the basis of the ISS (see Table 4.2) and genetic marker data from bone marrow plasma cells at diagnosis (Table 4.5).[4]

High-risk patients with ISS Stage II and III and t(4;14) or del(17p) – who represent up to 20% of newly diagnosed patients – have a predicted overall survival of 2 years.

Ultra-high-risk patients, with ISS stage III, high LDH levels and t(4;14) or del(17p) are unlikely to live for longer than 2 years from diagnosis without aggressive maintenance therapy.[5]

TABLE 4.5

Risk stratification and possible therapeutic questions within each risk category

	Ultra-high risk	High risk	Standard risk	Low risk
ISS stage	III + high LDH	II/III	III	I/II
Genetic risk factors	t(4;14) or del(17p)	t(4;14) or del(17p)	None	None
Median OS (years)	< 2	2	7	> 10
% of patients	20		60	20
Therapeutic questions	Novel approaches required to increase sustained clinical response (e.g. prolonged maintenance therapy or mAb-based combination therapies, or immunotherapy)		Investigate novel maintenance strategies to improve PFS and OS	Curative potential Reduce toxicity PS-tailored therapeutic approach

ISS, International Staging System; LDH, lactate dehydrogenase; mAb, monoclonal antibody; PFS, progression-free survival; PS, performance status; OS, overall survival.

Clinical trials to validate these risk groups and to identify therapeutic combinations that will improve outcomes for these patients are urgently needed.

Monitoring and response assessment

Monitoring. Patients being treated for myeloma should be assessed in clinic at least monthly, whereas patients who are 'off therapy' can be monitored less often. It is important to identify symptoms patients are experiencing, particularly fatigue, bone pain and infections, and any

side effects of ongoing or recently completed therapy. The following should be performed at each visit for patients receiving therapy:
- complete blood count
- bone, renal and liver biochemistry profiles
- serum and urine electrophoresis plus immunofixation
- sFLC assay.

Imaging may be required but should be limited to skeletal radiography or MRI/CT of areas with previous plasmacytomas or new areas of pain. If relapse is suspected, a full skeletal survey and MRI scan of the spine and pelvis is often required to assess skeletal damage or the presence of plasmacytomas.

Response assessment. The level of M protein in blood and urine can be used to assess response to treatment.[6] As Table 4.6 shows, the decrease in serum and urine M protein can characterize the level of response. Patients with complete disappearance of M protein in urine and serum by immunofixation and disappearance of plasmacytomas should undergo a bone marrow assessment to confirm complete response (CR; < 5% plasma cells). Patients in whom a reduction in plasmacytoma or M protein is not achieved should be considered refractory to treatment and switched to an alternative therapy (see Chapter 8).

More stringent criteria for response have been developed to reflect the improvements in response rates achieved with combinations of immunomodulatory drugs and proteasome inhibitors:
- stringent CR is defined as normalization of the sFLC ratio
- immunophenotypic CR is defined as absence of phenotypically aberrant clonal plasma cells in bone marrow, with a minimum of 1 million total bone marrow cells analyzed by multiparametric flow cytometry (with more than four colors)
- molecular CR is defined as CR plus negative allele-specific oligonucleotide polymerase chain reaction (ASO PCR), sensitivity 10^{-5}.

Monitoring for relapse. Patients who respond to therapy should be monitored for clinical or biochemical relapse off therapy or while on maintenance therapy.

TABLE 4.6

Criteria for assessing response to treatment

Response category	Examples
Stringent complete response (sCR)	CR as defined below, plus: • normal FLC ratio AND • absence of clonal cells in bone marrow by immunohistochemistry or immunofluorescence
Complete response (CR)	Negative immunofixation (serum and urine) and disappearance of any soft tissue plasmacytomas and ≤ 5% plasma cells in bone marrow
Very good partial response (VGPR)	Serum and urine M protein detectable by immunofixation but not on electrophoresis OR ≥ 90% serum M protein reduction and urine M protein < 100 mg/24 h
Partial response (PR)	≥ 50% serum M protein reduction and ≥ 90% urine M protein reduction to 200 mg/ 24 h (if serum/urine M protein is unmeasurable, ≥ 50% decrease in the difference between involved and uninvolved sFLC levels is required; if serum/urine M protein and sFLC are both unmeasurable, ≥ 50% reduction in plasma cells is required, provided baseline bone marrow plasma cell percentage is ≥ 30%) AND ≥ 50% reduction in the size of soft tissue plasmacytoma (if present at baseline)
Stable disease (SD)	Does not meet criteria for CR, VGPR, PR or progressive disease
Flow MRD-negative[†]	Absence of phenotypically aberrant clonal plasma cells by NGF on bone marrow aspirates (using a validated method with a sensitivity of ≥ 1 in 10^5 nucleated cells)
Sequencing MRD-negative[†]	Absence of clonal plasma cells by NGS on bone marrow aspirate; presence of a clone is defined as < 2 identical sequencing reads obtained after DNA sequencing of bone marrow aspirates (using a validated method with a sensitivity of ≥ 1 in 10^5 nucleated cells)

(CONTINUED OVERLEAF)

TABLE 4.6 (CONTINUED)
Criteria for assessing response to treatment

Response category	Examples
Imaging-positive MRD-negative[†]	MRD negativity as defined by NGF or NGS plus disappearance of every area of increased tracer uptake found at baseline or a preceding PET/CT, or decrease to less mediastinal blood pool SUV, or decrease to less than that of surrounding normal tissue
Sustained MRD-negative[†]	MRD negativity in the marrow (NGF, NGS, or both) and by imaging as defined below, confirmed minimum of 1 year apart
	Subsequent evaluations can be used to further specify the duration of negativity (e.g. MRD-negative at 5 years); the method used should be stated

*Not recommended as an indicator of response; stable disease (SD) is best described by providing time to progression estimates.
FLC, free light chain; MRD, minimal residual disease negative; NGF, next-generation flow cytometry; NGS, next-generation sequencing; sFLC, serum FLC; SUV, standardized uptake value.

- Clinical relapse is characterized by the reappearance of anemia, hypercalcemia, bone pain or bone lesions, renal impairment or a new plasmacytoma.
- Biochemical relapse is defined as a rise in serum/urine M protein without clinical symptoms; significant biochemical relapse is an indication to start anti-myeloma therapy.

Asymptomatic patients do not require routine imaging at follow-up unless they have signs of clinical or biochemical relapse. Bone marrow examination is recommended at relapse to identify any further clonal changes in the plasma cells, which may indicate a poor prognosis.

Minimal residual disease
Effective multidrug combinations for the first-line treatment of MM have significantly improved clinical outcomes over the last 5–10 years, and well over half of patients achieve CR. However, the presence of

more than 0.01% abnormal plasma cells is detected in most patients after treatment, referred to as minimal residual disease (MRD). Both the Spanish and UK Myeloma Research Alliances have shown that patients who achieve MRD negativity have better outcomes than patients with residual disease.[7] A number of techniques are available to measure MRD: quantitative ASO PCR, next-generation flow cytometry and next-generation VDJ sequencing using patient-specific primers.[8] These techniques have been refined in order to make them suitable for routine use. Table 4.6 includes the criteria for MRD depending on the technique used, defined by the IMWG.[6] The IMWG recommends that information on MRD is obtained after each treatment stage (e.g. after induction, high-dose therapy/ASCT, consolidation, maintenance) but MRD tests should only be initiated if complete response is suspected. All the categories of response and MRD require there to be no evidence of progressive or new bone

Key points – diagnosis, staging and monitoring of multiple myeloma

- Early diagnosis of symptomatic multiple myeloma (MM) is critical to optimize clinical outcome.
- Baseline tests should be performed at diagnosis and repeated at relapse.
- A combination of findings using both the International Staging System and genetic analysis has enabled risk stratification in patients with MM.
- The International Myeloma Working Group response criteria should be used to assess response.
- The development of new effective treatment has driven the development of more rigorous response criteria, such as 'stringent', 'immunophenotypic' and 'molecular' complete response. Patients with minimal residual disease (MRD) negativity have better outcomes than patients with MRD. MRD negativity is therefore likely to become the benchmark in clinical trials of new first-line treatments.

lesions if radiographic studies are performed. However, radiographic studies are not required to satisfy these response requirements except for the requirement of FDG PET if imaging MRD-negative status is reported. Achieving MRD negativity will be a new treatment goal in trials of treatments for newly diagnosed MM.

References

1. Dimopoulos M, Kyle R, Fernand JP et al. Consensus recommendations for standard investigative workup: report of the International Myeloma Workshop Consensus Panel 3. *Blood* 2011;117:4701–5.

2. Greipp PR, San Miguel J, Durie BG et al. International staging system for multiple myeloma. *J Clin Oncol* 2005;23:3412–20.

3. Palumbo A, Avet-Loiseau H, Oliva S et al. Revised International Staging System for Multiple Myeloma: A Report From International Myeloma Working Group. *J Clin Oncol* 2015;33: 2863–9.

4. Moreau P, Cavo M, Sonneveld P. Combination of international scoring system 3, high lactate dehydrogenase, and t(4;14) and/or del(17p) identifies patients with multiple myeloma (MM) treated with front-line autologous stem-cell transplantation at high risk of early MM progression-related death. *J Clin Oncol* 2014; 32:2173–80.

5. Nooka AK, Kaufman JL, Muppidi S et al. Consolidation and maintenance therapy with lenalidomide, bortezomib and dexamethasone (RVD) in high-risk myeloma patients. *Leukemia* 2014;28:690–3.

6. Kumar S, Paiva B, Anderson KC et al. International Myeloma Working Group consensus criteria for response and minimal residual disease assessment in multiple myeloma. *Lancet Oncol* 2016;17: e328–46.

7. Rawstron AC, Orfao A, Beksac M et al. Report of the European Myeloma Network on multiparametric flow cytometry in multiple myeloma and related disorders. *Haematologica* 2008;93:431–8.

8. Mailankody S, Korde N, Lesokhin AM et al. Minimal residual disease in multiple myeloma: bringing the bench to the bedside. *Nat Rev Clin Oncol* 2015;12:286–95.

5 Genetics and multiple myeloma

Importantly, not all patients who receive a pathological diagnosis of multiple myeloma (MM) have the same natural history or response to therapy. As different subsets of patients with MM are identified, it will become increasingly important – and possible – to tailor treatment to the individual patient, with the ultimate goal of achieving cure.

Genetic assessment
The following techniques are used together for the genetic assessment of patients with MM:[1]
- routine cytogenetics (Figure 5.1)
- fluorescence in situ hybridization (FISH) (see Figure 5.1)
- gene expression profiling (GEP)
- genome sequencing and mutational analysis.

Routine cytogenetics. Cytogenetic abnormalities are seen on routine karyotyping and are associated with high-risk disease because of increased plasma cell proliferation. Patients with hyperdiploidy on karyotyping (an increased number of odd-numbered chromosomes) generally have better outcomes than those whose disease is non-hyperdiploid.

FISH. Although routine karyotyping can identify 15% of high-risk myeloma cases, most patients have a 'normal' karyotype, whereas studies using FISH have shown that nearly all patients with MM have some level of genetic change (see Figure 5.1), and that this approach can distinguish between high- and low-risk disease (Figure 5.2). Del(17/17p), gain(1q) and translocations t(4;14), t(14;16) and t(14;20) are associated with poorer outcomes (Figure 5.3). Interestingly, FISH identifies del(13q) in more than 50% of newly diagnosed patients but it is only associated with adverse outcomes in the presence of del(17p) or t(4;14). These markers provide more prognostic information than is available from routine karyotyping.

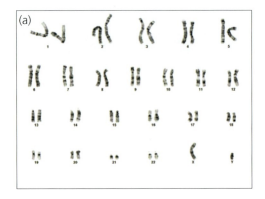

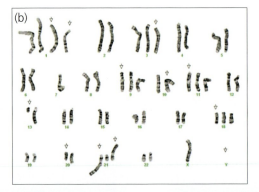

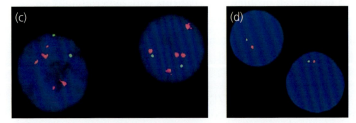

Figure 5.1 (a) Normal male XY karyotype. (b) Complex male XY karyotype of a myeloma patient, showing five copies of chromosome 1q (shown at chromosomes 1 and 21), del(13q14) and hyperdiploidy of mostly odd-numbered chromosomes (gains at 1, 3, 9, 11, 18 and 21). (c) FISH analysis showing gain of three copies of (1q21CKS1B), (1p32.3CDKN2C). (d) FISH analysis showing deletion 13 (13q14 D13S25), (13q34 LAMP). The deletion of both FISH markers makes it look like monosomy 13; however, karyotype (b) shows that part of chromosome 13 is retained just below the centromere. FISH, fluorescence in situ hybridization.

Genetics and multiple myeloma

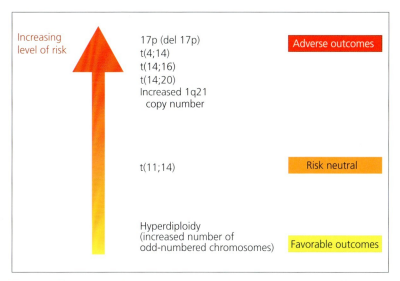

Figure 5.2 Relationships between genetic abnormalities, identified by fluorescence in situ hybridization (FISH), and clinical outcomes in multiple myeloma.

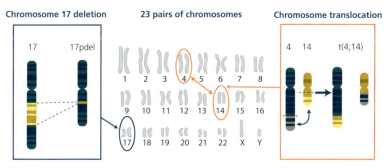

Figure 5.3 Mechanisms of genetic abnormalities in multiple myeloma.

The presence of genetic aberrations is not important in the choice of induction therapy; however, many groups are now tailoring maintenance therapy according to genetic abnormalities identified on FISH.

It should be noted that the identification of genetic changes using FISH requires myeloma cells to be isolated or identified with cytoplasmic immunoglobulin (cIG) staining, which uses a fluorescent probe with light chains to identify the tumor cells prior to FISH.

However, many laboratories perform FISH testing on the whole bone marrow aspirate, and may therefore be under-reporting the presence of genetic abnormalities.

The revised ISS includes genetic abnormalities identified by FISH (see Table 4.4, page 44).

Gene expression profiling. Although FISH testing has allowed clinicians to identify subsets of patients with different genetic changes, not all patients with a given genetic abnormality will have the same outcome. GEP has therefore been used to gain greater insight into tumor biology. Several different GEP-based assessments have been used to stratify risk and determine prognosis. At least four profiles are associated with poor-risk MM in clinical trials but there is no overlap between the genes in each case, which suggests that the differences in predictive power between profiles may be related to the treatments used in the respective trials.[2] Nevertheless, GEP-based risk assessment is useful to identify differences between individual patients and can provide additional information that may reflect gene function. To date, no single profile has been adopted into routine clinical practice.

Sequencing and mutational analysis. The most recent approach to identifying genetic differences between patients with MM involves the use of genome sequencing, either in a targeted fashion, focusing on a small number of known potential mutations, or with a broader whole-genome approach. In initial studies, the most frequent mutations affected the *NRAS* and *KRAS* genes, and mutations affecting nuclear factor (NF)-κB were also common.[3] It is worth noting that 4% of patients had *BRAF* mutations, which can potentially be targeted using agents used in colorectal cancer and melanoma; indeed, there have been a few reports of the successful use of BRAF-targeted agents in the treatment of patients with refractory MM with a mutation in this gene.[4] However, there may be subsets of patients who do not respond to BRAF inhibitor monotherapy although other mutations may provide opportunities for targeted treatment.

Several groups are now investigating the use of mutational analysis to predict response to therapy. One study from the UK Medical Research Council has identified 'good' and 'poor' risk mutations in patients receiving alkylating agent-based therapies. Mutations known to be associated with poor outcomes include those associated with DNA repair, which suggests that mutation-driven approaches may be treatment-specific.[5] This in turn implies that mutational analysis needs broader validation across a range of treatment approaches before it can be routinely applied in clinical practice.

Genetic assessment after treatment and at relapse

Myeloma patients present with multiple clones, and it is important to consider how the presence of intraclonal heterogeneity affects treatment,[6] as clonal tiding (changes in the subclonal structure over time) and development of resistance make treatment planning in the relapsed setting quite challenging. Genetic assessment of plasma cells after treatment can be technically demanding, and FISH failure rates are higher in studies of patients with relapsed disease;[7] however, clonal tiding can result in newer clones that can help to direct therapy.[8]

Key points – genetics and multiple myeloma

- Risk assessment and identification of different subgroups of patients with MM based on genetics remains a key goal, as personalized treatment becomes more important.
- Genetic characterization using fluorescence in situ hybridization (FISH) has been incorporated into the revised International Staging System (rISS) risk stratification. While this does not affect the choice of initial therapy, it is important when planning maintenance therapy.
- In patients with relapsed disease, genetic analyses may be useful to inform decisions about treatment.
- Targeted mutational analysis may be useful in the setting of minimal residual disease to better define how to eliminate the remaining clone, thereby improving treatment outcomes.

In patients with minimal residual disease (see page 48) following therapy, the analysis of clonal structures using next-generation sequencing will help build strategies for tumor eradication and help personalize therapy in this setting – this is likely to become an area of significant research interest over the next few years.

References

1. Avet-Loiseau H. Role of genetics in prognostication in myeloma. Best practice and research. *Clin Haematol* 2007;20:625–35.

2. Chng WJ, Dispenzieri A, Chim CS et al. IMWG consensus on risk stratification in multiple myeloma. *Leukemia* 2014;28:269–77.

3. Chapman MA, Lawrence MS, Keats JJ et al. Initial genome sequencing and analysis of multiple myeloma. *Nature* 2011;471:467–72.

4. Andrulis M, Lehners N, Capper D et al. Targeting the BRAF V600E mutation in multiple myeloma. *Cancer Discovery* 2013;3:862–9.

5. Walker BA, Boyle EM, Wardell CP et al. Mutational spectrum, copy number changes, and outcome: results of a sequencing study of patients with newly diagnosed myeloma. *J Clin Oncol* 2015;33:3911–20.

6. Morgan GJ, Walker BA, Davies FE. The genetic architecture of multiple myeloma. *Nat Rev Cancer* 2012;12:335–48.

7. Cook G, Williams C, Brown JM et al. High-dose chemotherapy plus autologous stem-cell transplantation as consolidation therapy in patients with relapsed multiple myeloma after previous autologous stem-cell transplantation (NCRI Myeloma X Relapse [Intensive trial]): a randomised, open-label, phase 3 trial. *Lancet Oncol* 2014;15:874–85.

8. Smith D, Stephenson C, Percy L et al. Cohort analysis of FISH testing of CD138(+) cells in relapsed multiple myeloma: implications for prognosis and choice of therapy. *Br J Haematol* 2015;171:881–3.

6 Treatment of newly diagnosed multiple myeloma

The treatment of newly diagnosed multiple myeloma (MM) involves induction therapy to reduce the tumor burden and improve symptoms. This typically involves two- or three-drug combinations of an immunomodulatory drug [IMiD], such as thalidomide or lenalidomide (an analog of thalidomide that is more potent and less toxic), a proteasome inhibitor (PI) such as bortezomib or carfilzomib, and a steroid (often dexamethasone).

Where appropriate, this is followed by consolidation therapy, which involves high-dose therapy and autologous stem cell transplantation (ASCT) (Figure 6.1).[1] Consolidation is followed with maintenance therapy.

The choice of treatment strategy and induction regimen is of utmost importance, and should be considered carefully when initiating therapy; it is incumbent on treating clinicians to treat to maximal response, and to consider long-term treatment strategies. Median survival for many patients now exceeds 8–10 years.

When to start

The criteria for starting induction therapy are largely based on clinical assessment of myeloma symptoms resulting from end organ damage, defined according to the CRAB criteria (hyperCalcemia, Renal insufficiency, Anemia and Bone disease). The presence of any of these signs indicates symptomatic myeloma, and that therapy should be started. The International Myeloma Working Group (IMWG) has recently extended the definition of symptomatic MM to include histological and monoclonal protein criteria, including any of the following (the so-called SLiM CRAB; see page 25):
- 60% or more abnormal plasma cells in the bone marrow
- serum free light chain (sFLC) ratio above 100
- more than one focal bone lesion on MRI.

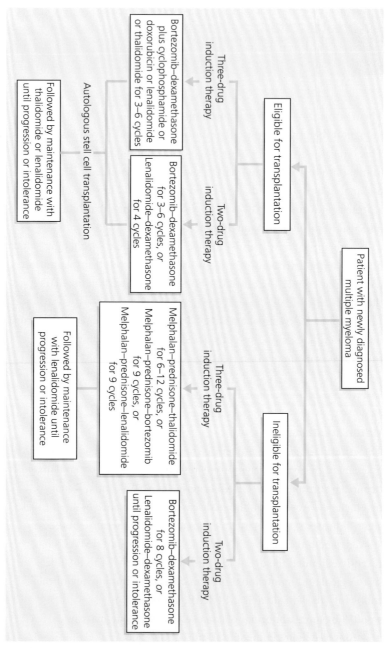

Figure 6.1 A suggested approach to the treatment of patients with newly diagnosed multiple myeloma.[19]

Patients meeting any of these criteria are considered to be at very high risk of rapid progression to symptomatic MM and are thus eligible for treatment.

Smoldering myeloma. Recent studies have investigated the effect of treating patients with high- or intermediate-risk smoldering myeloma (for whom the benefits of early therapy have hitherto been unclear). A small randomized trial found that, compared with observation alone, lenalidomide plus dexamethasone improved time to development of symptomatic MM and overall survival (OS) in asymptomatic patients with a high risk of progression.[2] Further studies to establish the benefits of early treatment of smoldering myeloma are in progress; in the meantime, patients who do not fit the revised definition of symptomatic MM (see page 25) should not be treated, except in the context of a clinical trial.

Transplant-eligible patients

High-dose induction therapy (Tables 6.1 and 6.2) followed by ASCT is standard treatment for patients who are fit and have reasonable performance status (i.e. PS < 2).[9] In most European centers, patients up to age 65 years are considered eligible for ASCT, whereas most US transplant centers will consider ASCT for patients up to 78 years of age, provided their performance status is acceptable. The dose of melphalan may be reduced in older patients.

Eligible patients should be referred to an appropriate transplant or myeloma center early in their treatment for consideration of stem cell collection and transplantation. Patients undergo 3–6 cycles of induction therapy to reduce the tumor burden and symptoms before stem cell collection.

Three- versus two-drug regimens. Three-drug regimens are associated with a higher objective response rate and depth of response (i.e. a higher complete response [CR] rate) than two-drug regimens, and investigators now largely agree that the benefit outweighs the risk of toxicity. Hence, induction therapy with triple-drug regimens comprising a PI, IMiD and a steroid, such as bortezomib–thalidomide–

TABLE 6.1

Induction therapy combinations (supported by Phase III data)

Regimen (n)	Post-induction CR/nCR	≥ VGPR	ORR
Bortezomib-based regimens			
BD (240) vs	14.8	37.7	78.5
VAD (242)	6.4	15.1	62.8
p value	0.004	< 0.001	< 0.001
Harosseau[3]			
VTD (236) vs	31	62	93
TD (238)	11	28	79
p value	< 0.0001	< 0.001	< 0.001
Cavo[4]			
BAD (413) vs	11	42	78
VAD (414)	5	14	54
p value	< 0.001	< 0.001	< 0.001
Sonneveld[5]			
VTD (100) vs	31	49	88
VD (99)	22	36	81
p value	0.15	0.05	0.19
Moreau[6]			
Lenalidomide-based regimens			
RD (223) vs	2.3	42.1	79
Rd (222)	1.4	23.6	68.3
p value		< 0.0001	0.008
Rajkumar[7]			

Response rates are percentages of patients. *Best response (not post-transplant).
A, doxorubicin (adriamycin); B, bortezomib; D, dexamethasone;
Rd, lenalidomide with low-dose dexamethasone; RD: lenalidomide with high-dose dexamethasone; T, thalidomide; V, vincristine.
CR/nCR, complete response/near complete response; ORR, objective response rate; OS, overall survival; PFS, progression-free survival; VGPR, very good partial response; y, years.

Post-transplantation				
CR	≥ VGPR	ORR	PFS (%)	OS (%)
35	54.3	80.3	36	81.4 (3y)
18.4	37.2	77.1	29.7	77.4 (3y)
< 0.001	< 0.001	0.401	0.06	0.5
52	79	93	68 (3y)	86 (3y)
31	58	84	56 (3y)	84 (3y)
< 0.001	< 0.001	< 0.001	0.005	0.3
36	76	90	35	61 (5y)
24	56	83	28	55 (5y)
< 0.001	< 0.001	0.002	0.002	0.11
29	77	89	26	
31	58	86	30	
0.77	0.02	0.54	0.22	
5	50*	81		92 (3y)
4	40*	70		
0.04	0.04	0.009		

dexamethasone (VTD), is now standard practice for most transplant-eligible patients. The benefits of triple-drug compared with double-drug regimens are probably most important for high-risk patients such as those with *p53* deletion and t(4;14) translocation, but this approach is also beneficial for standard-risk patients. Recent data from the

TABLE 6.2

Induction therapy combinations (supported by Phase II data)

Regimen (n)	ORR	CR + nCR	≥ VGPR
VRD (66)	100	44	74
VCD bi-weekly (33)	88	39	61
VCD weekly (30)	93	43	60
CRD (53)	98	62	81
IRD[8]	92	35	58

All response rates are percentages of patient.
CRD, carfilzomib, lenalidomide, dexamethasone; IRD, ixazomib, lenalidomide, dexamethasone; VCD, bortezomib, cyclophosphamide, dexamethasone; VRD, bortezomib, lenalidomide, dexamethasone.
CR, complete response; nCR, near complete response; ORR, objective response rate; VGPR, very good partial response (includes patients with no measurable M protein who have not had bone marrow assessments to confirm CR/nCR status).

SWOG trial demonstrating the survival benefit of adding bortezomib to lenalidomide–dexamethasone (VRD vs RD) has now solidified the role of three-drug regimens for fit patients.[10] Furthermore, the recently published IFM (Intergroupe Francophone du Myelome) trial, which demonstrated the superiority of VTD over VCD (bortezomib–cyclophosphamide–dexamethasone) has relegated use of alkylating agent-based induction therapy to second choice behind the IMiD–PI–steroid triplets.[6] VRD is now widely used in the USA for induction therapy, having been initially explored by the Dana–Farber Cancer Institute and IFM.[11,12] Carfilzomib in combination with lenalidomide and dexamethasone has shown significantly high response rates in patients with newly diagnosed MM,[13] and is now being compared with VRD in a Phase III trial.

Trials of four-drug regimens comprising an IMiD, PI, steroid and alkylating agent have also been reported, with significantly high response rates and acceptable tolerability.

Goals of induction therapy. A major goal is to achieve a very good partial response (VGPR) or better, and the induction regimen with the highest likelihood of achieving this should be chosen. Patients who do not achieve a VGPR following induction therapy do not require a second round of induction therapy and should proceed to stem cell collection and ASCT. One exception to this is patients in whom the maximum response is less than a partial response (PR), who should be considered to have primary refractory myeloma and may benefit from an alternative regimen prior to high-dose melphalan.[14]

The role of ASCT in newly diagnosed MM has been questioned in view of the very high CR rates that are achieved with modern three- and four-drug induction regimens; however, significant survival benefits have been shown with transplantation. For example, a study that compared lenalidomide plus dexamethasone induction therapy followed by transplantation versus low-dose melphalan with lenalidomide showed longer progression-free survival (PFS) and OS in the patients who underwent ASCT, even though the CR rate was the same in both groups; this possibly reflects the higher proportion of patients with no minimal residual disease in the transplant group.[15] A further trial that compared lenalidomide versus high- or low-dose dexamethasone reported longer OS in patients who proceeded to ASCT than in those who did not. Thus, there remains considerable evidence favoring the use of ASCT, even with the new induction regimens.

The timing of transplantation has been investigated in a number of retrospective studies, and is being further investigated in prospective trials. While some data indicate no difference between early or late transplantation (i.e. less than versus more than a year from diagnosis) in terms of OS, even with novel agents, the standard recommendation continues to be that most patients should proceed to early transplant, with the intention of maximizing the duration of first remission.

The use of tandem ASCT has decreased significantly in recent years in favor of consolidation or maintenance therapies. By contrast, a second transplant following relapse is becoming increasingly common, provided that the duration of the response to first transplant is at least 2 years. It is therefore important to obtain sufficient cells for multiple transplants at the initial harvest.

Transplant-ineligible patients

Ineligibility for transplant is not clearly defined but most clinicians agree that performance status or frailty index is a better determinant than age when considering the best treatment approach. In an elderly patient with MM, frailty, ongoing comorbidities and disability should all be assessed before choosing a therapy. The Eastern Cooperative Oncology Group (ECOG) performance status is the most widely used assessment of functional status and is often used to guide therapy; however, this is less suitable for the geriatric population: 9–38% of elderly patients (> 70 years) with a good performance status (< 2) are partially or fully dependent on others to carry out ordinary activities such as household tasks and personal care.

Many prognostic indices for the elderly are available that incorporate age, comorbidity or both; the Charlson comorbidity index is most frequently used in patients with cancer and has been validated in myelodysplastic syndrome. To date, no myeloma studies have prospectively assessed outcomes in patients with varying abilities and comorbidities. Until such data become available, chemotherapy doses are often attenuated empirically, and patients require close follow-up. Clinical judgment, discussion with the multidisciplinary team and consideration of patient choice are all important.

While the combination of melphalan with prednisone (MP) has been the gold-standard treatment for over 40 years, lenalidomide- and bortezomib-based induction regimens are increasingly being used, even for elderly patients (Table 6.3). These regimens have comparable efficacy to melphalan-based regimens and are well tolerated. Importantly, the FIRST (Frontline Investigation of Revlimid and Dexamethasone versus Standard Thalidomide) trial showed that patients receiving continuous treatment with lenalidomide and low-dose dexamethasone had significantly better PFS than those receiving lenalidomide–dexamethasone only for 72 cycles or a melphalan–prednisone–thalidomide (MPT) combination, and significantly longer OS. This study represented a paradigm shift in the treatment of MM, as it provided conclusive evidence that continuous non-melphalan induction therapy can have a positive effect on both duration of response and OS.

TABLE 6.3

Induction regimens for elderly patients

	VISTA[16]		IFM 99–06[17]		FIRST[18]		Meta-analysis[19]	MM-015[20]	
	VMP	MP	MPT	MP	Rd	MPT	MPT vs MP	MPR-R	MP
ORR* (%)	71	35	76	35	75	62	3.39[†]	77	49
CR (%)	30	4	13	2	15	9	NR	18	5
Median TTP (mo)	24		16.6	NR	NR	32.5	23.9	NR	NR
HR	0.48				0.68				
(*p* value)	(< 0.001)				(< 0.001)				
Median PFS (mo)	NR		NR	27.5	17.8	25.5	21.2	31	13
HR			0.45		0.72			0.398	
(*p* value)			(< 0.0001)		(< 0.0001)			(< 0.0000001)	
Median OS (mo)	56.4		43.1	51.6	33.2	59%[‡]	51%	NR	NR
HR	0.695		0.56		0.78				
(*p* value)	(0.0004)		(0.002)		(0.02)				

*CR + PR, assessed by European Group for Blood and Marrow Transplantation criteria.
[†]Pooled odds ratio in favor of MPT. [‡]% at 4 years.
CR, complete response; d, low-dose dexamethasone; FIRST, Frontline Investigation of Revlimid and Dexamethasone versus Standard Thalidomide; HR, hazard ratio; IFM, Intergroupe Francophone du Myelome; M, melphalan; MM, multiple myeloma; mo, months; NR, not reported; ORR, objective response rate; OS, overall survival; P, prednisone; R, lenalidomide; -R, lenalidomide maintenance; T, thalidomide, V, bortezomib; TTP, time to progression; VISTA, Velcade as Initial Standard Therapy in Multiple Myeloma.

The current standard of care for transplant-ineligible patients includes lenalidomide plus low-dose dexamethasone, as it is safe, well tolerated and easy to administer to frail patients. Alternatives involving the addition of a monoclonal antibody or the oral PI ixazomib to lenalidomide plus low-dose dexamethasone are being studied.

High-risk patients

The optimal management of patients who are considered to be high risk at presentation is still being explored. It is generally accepted that combinations that include either bortezomib or lenalidomide are needed, but there is no consensus regarding the optimal induction regimen. A trial evaluating the addition of bortezomib to thalidomide and dexamethasone (VTD vs TD) and a chemotherapy-based approach found that response rates were highest with the VTD regimen. This is further supported by the very high objective response rate with VRD in both standard- and high-risk myeloma patients. However, achieving a CR is not sufficient in this setting, and prolonged maintenance is needed to maximize the duration of response. There is evidence that both PFS and OS may be improved by bortezomib compared with thalidomide maintenance therapy in high-risk patients.

Similarly, the use of VRD after ASCT may ameliorate the poor prognosis associated with t(4;14), and may improve outcomes for highest-risk patients when used as part of a planned treatment strategy.[21] Further studies are needed to determine the optimal duration of maintenance therapy, and to evaluate the use of combination approaches for high-risk patients.

The IMWG has recently developed a consensus statement for the treatment of high-risk patients, presented in Table 6.4.[22]

TABLE 6.4

Consensus statement developed by the International Working Group for Myeloma for the treatment of patients with cytogenetic high-risk disease[22]

Thalidomide	• Does not abrogate the adverse effect of t(4;14), t(14;16), t(14;20), and del(17) or del(17p) and gain(1q) CA
	• Conclusive data for elderly or frail patients are not available
Bortezomib	• Partly overcomes the adverse effect of t(4;14) and possibly del(17p) on CR, PFS, and OS
	• There is no effect in t(4;14) combined with del(17p) in TE patients
	• VMP may partly restore PFS in HR cytogenetics in non-TE patients

(CONTINUED)

Lenalidomide	• Partly improves the adverse effect of t(4;14) and del(17p) on PFS, but not OS, in TE patients
	• No data suggesting that the drug may improve outcome with HR cytogenetics in non-TE patients
Pomalidomide	• Pomalidomide with dexamethasone showed promising results in RRMM with del(17p)
PI plus lenalidomide	• Combining a PI with lenalidomide and dexamethasone greatly reduces the adverse effect of t(4;14) and del(17p) on PFS in NDMM
	• Carfilzomib with lenalidomide and dexamethasone seems effective in patients with HR cytogenetics. However, with exception of ASPIRE and TOURMALINE, most data were from non-randomized studies and long-term follow-up has not been reported
	• The group advises treating NDMM patients with HR cytogenetics with a PI in combination with lenalidomide or pomalidomide and dexamethasone
HDT + ASCT	• HDT with ASCT is standard therapy for TE patients with NDMM, contributing to improved outcome across prognostic groups
	• Double HDT/ASCT combined with bortezomib may improve PFS in patients with t(4;14), del(17p) or both.
	• Although results from stratified randomized trials are not yet available, HDT plus double ASCT is recommended for patients with HR cytogenetics
Allo-SCT	• Allo-SCT or tandem auto-allo-SCT may improve PFS in patients with t(4;14) or del(17p); results are better at early stages of the disease
	• The novel treatments may challenge the role of allo-SCT; use should be restricted to clinical trials

Allo-SCT, allogeneic stem cell transplantation; ASCT, autologous stem cell transplantation; CA, chromosomal abnormalities; CR, complete response; HDT, high-dose therapy; HR, high-risk; NDDM, newly diagnosed multiple myeloma; OS, overall survival; PFS, progression-free survival; PI, proteasome inhibitor; TE, transplant eligible.

Key points – Treatment of newly diagnosed multiple myeloma

- Patients with smoldering myeloma who meet new histological and monoclonal protein criteria (established by the International Myeloma Working Group) are considered to be at very high risk of rapid progression to symptomatic multiple myeloma (MM) and are thus eligible for treatment.
- Induction therapy with triple-drug regimens comprising a proteasome inhibitor (PI), an immunomodulatory drug [IMiD] and a steroid, followed by early transplant and maintenance, is now the standard of care for most transplant-eligible patients.
- The use of combination therapy, and attempts to prolong the duration of the first remission, are priorities.
- Despite the high complete response rates seen with induction therapies, there is considerable evidence that autologous stem cell transplantation provides additional benefit.
- Continuous therapy with lenalidomide plus dexamethasone has emerged as the standard of care for transplant-ineligible patients.
- The growing focus on risk stratification, particularly in the maintenance setting, will help to improve the rate of sustained complete response, making the prospect of cure more realistic.
- The optimal management of patients who are considered to be high risk at presentation is still being explored.

References

1. Palumbo A and Anderson K. Multiple myeloma. *New Engl J Med* 2011;36:1046–60.

2. Mateos MV, Hernandez MT, Giraldo P et al. Lenalidomide plus dexamethasone for high-risk smoldering multiple myeloma. *N Engl J Med* 2013;369:438–47.

3. Harousseau JL, Attal M, Avet-Loiseau H et al. Bortezomib plus dexamethasone is superior to vincristine plus doxorubicin plus dexamethasone as induction treatment prior to autologous stem-cell transplantation in newly diagnosed multiple myeloma: results of the IFM 2005-01 phase III trial. *J Clin Oncol* 2010;28:4621–9.

4. Cavo M, Tacchetti P, Patriarca F et al. Bortezomib with thalidomide plus dexamethasone compared with thalidomide plus dexamethasone as induction therapy before, and consolidation therapy after, double autologous stem-cell transplantation in newly diagnosed multiple myeloma: a randomised phase 3 study. *Lancet* 2010;376:2075–85.

5. Sonneveld P, Schmidt-Wolf IG, van der Holt B et al. Bortezomib induction and maintenance treatment in patients with newly diagnosed multiple myeloma: results of the randomized phase III HOVON-65/ GMMG-HD4 trial. *J Clin Oncol* 2012;30:2946–55.

6. Moreau P, Avet-Loiseau H, Facon T et al. Bortezomib plus dexamethasone versus reduced-dose bortezomib, thalidomide plus dexamethasone as induction treatment before autologous stem cell transplantation in newly diagnosed multiple myeloma. *Blood* 2011;118:5752–8; quiz 982.

7. Rajkumar SV, Jacobus S, Callander NS et al. Lenalidomide plus high-dose dexamethasone versus lenalidomide plus low-dose dexamethasone as initial therapy for newly diagnosed multiple myeloma: an open-label randomised controlled trial. *Lancet Oncol* 2010;11:29–37.

8. Kumar SK, Berdeja JG, Niesvizky R et al. Safety and tolerability of ixazomib, an oral proteasome inhibitor, in combination with lenalidomide and dexamethasone in patients with previously untreated multiple myeloma: an open-label phase 1/2 study. *Lancet Oncol* 2014;15:1503–12.

9. Cavo M, Rajkumar SV, Palumbo A et al. International Myeloma Working Group consensus approach to the treatment of multiple myeloma patients who are candidates for autologous stem cell transplantation. *Blood* 2011;117:6063–73.

10. Durie D, Hoering A, Rajkumar SV et al, Bortezomib, lenalidomide and dexamethasone vs. lenalidomide and dexamethasone in patients (pts) with previously untreated multiple myeloma without an intent for immediate autologous stem cell transplant (ASCT): results of the randomized phase III trial SWOG S0777. *Blood* 2015;126:25.

11. Richardson PG, Weller E, Lonial S et al. Lenalidomide, bortezomib, and dexamethasone combination therapy in patients with newly diagnosed multiple myeloma. *Blood* 2010;116:679–86.

12. Roussel M, Lauwers-Cances V, Robillard N et al. Front-line transplantation program with lenalidomide, bortezomib, and dexamethasone combination as induction and consolidation followed by lenalidomide maintenance in patients with multiple myeloma: a phase II study by the Intergroupe Francophone du Myelome. *J Clin Oncol* 2014;32:2712–7.

13. Jakubowiak AJ, Dytfeld D, Griffith KA et al. A phase 1/2 study of carfilzomib in combination with lenalidomide and low-dose dexamethasone as a frontline treatment for multiple myeloma. *Blood* 2012;120:1801–9.

14. Vij R, Kumar S, Zhang MJ et al. Impact of pretransplant therapy and depth of disease response before autologous transplantation for multiple myeloma. *Biol Blood Marrow Transplant* 2015;21: 335–41.

15. Palumbo A, Cavallo F, Gay F et al. Autologous transplantation and maintenance therapy in multiple myeloma. *N Engl J Med* 2014;371:895–905.

16. San Miguel JF, Schlag R, Khuageva NK et al. Bortezomib plus melphalan and prednisone for initial treatment of multiple myeloma. *N Engl J Med* 2008;359:906–17.

17. Facon T, Mary JY, Hulin C et al. Melphalan and prednisone plus thalidomide versus melphalan and prednisone alone or reduced-intensity autologous stem cell transplantation in elderly patients with multiple myeloma (IFM 99-06): a randomised trial. *Lancet* 2007;370:1209–18.

18. Benboubker L, Dimopoulos MA, Dispenzieri A et al. Lenalidomide and dexamethasone in transplant-ineligible patients with myeloma. *N Engl J Med* 2014;371:906–17.

19. Kapoor P, Rajkumar SV, Dispenzieri et al. Melphalan and prednisone versus melphalan, prednisone and thalidomide for elderly and/or transplant ineligible patients with multiple myeloma: a meta-analysis. *Leukemia* 2011;2:689–96.

20. Palumbo A, Hajek R, Delforge M et al. Continuous lenalidomide treatment for newly diagnosed multiple myeloma. *N Engl J Med* 2012;366:1759–69.

21. Nooka AK, Kaufman JL, Muppidi S et al. Consolidation and maintenance therapy with lenalidomide, bortezomib and dexamethasone (RVD) in high-risk myeloma patients. *Leukemia* 2014;28:690–3.

22. Sonneveld P, Avet-Loiseau H, Lonial S et al. Treatment of multiple myeloma with high-risk cytogenetics: a consensus of the International Myeloma Working Group. *Blood* 2016;127:2955–62.

7 Stem cell transplantation in multiple myeloma

High-dose therapy (HDT) and stem cell transplantation (SCT) improves the duration and depth of response and overall survival (OS), and is the standard of care for eligible patients. Patients first undergo induction chemotherapy (see Chapter 6) to reduce the symptom/disease burden, ahead of conditioning HDT and SCT. The benefit of autologous SCT (ASCT) has been questioned in view of the high complete response (CR) rates achieved with modern induction regimens; however, trials continue to demonstrate benefits of ASCT in terms of both duration of response and OS.

Conditioning regimens

The standard approach for conditioning before ASCT (i.e. preparative chemotherapy) in multiple myeloma (MM) has traditionally been melphalan 200 mg/m^2; several trials have explored alternative conditioning regimens with and without melphalan but have largely found these to have similar benefits but with greater toxicity.[1,2]

Several studies have investigated the use of novel agents in conditioning regimens. A Phase I trial found that bortezomib could be safely combined with standard-dose melphalan; the optimal treatment sequence was a single dose of bortezomib after administration of melphalan, in order to optimize the potential synergy between the two agents.[3,4] Similar results were obtained in a further trial, in which patients received two doses of bortezomib before administration of melphalan and two afterwards. Both trials suggested that the CR rate after ASCT was higher when bortezomib was added to the conditioning regimen; further trials are needed to explore this approach further.

Age and outcome after transplantation

HDT followed by ASCT is generally considered for patients who are young and fit, and hence arbitrary age thresholds have been applied when considering eligibility for such treatment. In Europe, this threshold is generally considered to be 65 years. In the USA, by contrast, performance status is more important than age, and Medicare covers ASCT for patients with MM up to 78 years of age.

Several studies have reported benefits with HDT in older patients, including one analysis which suggested that patients over 65 years of age benefited as much as younger patients.[5] Indeed, there is evidence that selected elderly patients with good performance status have better outcomes than matched patients who do not undergo ASCT. This suggests that, while not all elderly patients are suitable for ASCT, age alone is not a sufficient criterion for exclusion. In older patients (> 70 years), lower doses of melphalan (140 mg/m^2) should be used to minimize toxicity. Dose-reduced ASCT has also been shown to be safe in patients with MM and renal impairment.[6]

Role of induction therapy

In the past, ASCT was used to achieve CR following relatively ineffective induction regimens (steroids or alkylating agent-based therapy), and the survival benefit associated with ASCT was partly correlated with a higher post-transplant CR rate. However, CR can now be achieved with four cycles of induction regimens using agents such as bortezomib, lenalidomide, thalidomide or carfilzomib, raising the question of whether ASCT continues to offer benefit.

Several trials have addressed this question both indirectly and directly. In a trial conducted by the Italian Myeloma Group, the addition of bortezomib to thalidomide–dexamethasone induction therapy (i.e. VTD vs TD) was associated with an almost twofold increase in the proportion of patients achieving a very good partial response (VGPR) or better and an improvement in post-transplant progression-free survival (PFS). A further study reported a significant improvement in OS and PFS favoring patients who underwent early ASCT compared with those who opted not to proceed to ASCT, even though the pre-transplant CR rate was higher in the latter group.

More recent trials of induction with lenalidomide and low-dose dexamethasone (Rd) followed by either ASCT or consolidation therapy with melphalan or cyclophosphamide plus Rd showed improvements in PFS and OS in patients undergoing early transplantation compared with those who received consolidation therapy, even though the CR rates were similar in the two arms.

Such studies show that HDT confers significant survival benefits even after a major response is achieved with modern induction regimens. The effect appears at least in part to increase the depth of response and to achieve minimal residual disease (MRD)-negativity in a higher proportion of patients. MRD-negativity by flow cytometry (see Table 4.6, page 47) was associated with significantly improved PFS in both the MRC and Spanish trials.

Allogeneic stem cell transplantation

To date, randomized clinical trials have not shown any significant benefit of allogeneic SCT (allo-SCT) for standard- or high-risk patients with newly diagnosed MM, although this approach is still being evaluated in younger patients. Increased treatment-related mortality associated with the older age of the average patient with MM is thought to limit the overall efficacy and safety of allo-SCT.[7,8] Similarly, the role of allo-SCT as salvage therapy for patients with relapsed or refractory myeloma remains unclear, in part because the outcomes for patients with relapsed MM have improved significantly with the advent of new drugs.

Patients with standard-risk MM (as assessed by genetic evaluation [see Chapter 5]) have a long median OS after relapse (5–7 years), whereas those with genetic abnormalities associated with poor risk are likely to have proliferative disease that is too severe for allo-SCT to be of any benefit. Although a small proportion of patients may derive long-term benefit from allo-SCT, the mortality and morbidity resulting from acute or chronic graft versus host disease strongly outweigh the benefits; the probability of benefit from allo-SCT in a patient with aggressive relapse, or among patients with high-risk MM, also remains unproven. Notwithstanding the high risk of transplant-related mortality, allo-SCT may be considered in high-risk patients who achieve a good response with salvage therapy, preferably in the setting of a clinical trial and using newer agents such as bortezomib for graft modulation after transplantation.[9–12] However, allo-SCT should not be routinely considered for patients with relapsing or refractory MM outside the context of well-designed clinical trials.

Cellular therapy

Several cellular-based treatments in addition to allo-SCT are being investigated in MM (Table 7.1).

Natural killer cell-based cellular infusion has been used in patients undergoing haploidentical transplantation (a haploidentical related donor is usually a 50% match to the recipient and may be their parent, sibling or child) for other malignancies, and is being evaluated in MM as part of a therapeutic strategy for patients who are receiving bortezomib-based salvage therapy[13–15] following promising preclinical work. The use of antibodies directed to killer cell immunoglobulin-like receptors (KIRs) on natural killer cells is also being investigated, with the aim of inducing anti-tumor activity in endogenous natural killer cells.[16,17] Preclinical data suggest that a combination of lenalidomide with an antibody that blocks KIR–ligand interaction induces significant responses in a murine model, although clinical trials to date have not shown significant anti-tumor activity.

Chimeric antigen receptor technology (CART) has also been investigated in MM. CART refers to the fusion of the antigen-recognizing portion of a monoclonal antibody with the signaling elements of T cells. These molecules are genetically grafted into T lymphocytes, allowing them to bind to tumor surface antigens in a

TABLE 7.1

Cellular-based therapies being investigated in multiple myeloma

- Natural-killer cell-based cellular infusion
- Chimeric antigen receptor T cells (CART)
- Dendritic cell vaccines

major histocompatibility complex (MHC)-independent fashion and promote T cell co-stimulation. CART has been developed to redirect and enhance T-cell effector functions by activating their cytotoxic pathways against the malignant cells. Most studies have used the CD19 construct, which has been successful in patients with acute lymphoblastic leukemia; however, data for MM are limited. Additional potential strategies include the use of the cell surface CS1 antigen or B cell maturation antigen as therapeutic targets, which may be better targets in MM than CD19 because they are expressed to greater extents on the cell surface.

Dendritic cell vaccines provide another potential approach to immunotherapy, and both whole-cell and antigen-specific vaccines are being evaluated in Phase I or combination trials in patients with relapsed or smoldering myeloma. Tumor vaccines are designed to re-educate the host immunity to recognize myeloma cells as foreign by expanding tumor-specific T cells and creating long-term memory to prevent recurrence. This approach therefore aims to enhance innate immunity to produce an anti-tumor effect.

Key points – Stem cell transplantation in multiple myeloma

- High-dose therapy followed by autologous stem cell transplantation (SCT) remains a standard approach in the treatment of suitable patients with newly diagnosed myeloma.
- The benefits of autologous SCT may be enhanced by better induction and maintenance regimens to achieve low levels of minimal residual disease (MRD) or MRD negativity.
- The use of allogeneic SCT in myeloma remains experimental.
- Cellular therapies that enhance innate immunity may be an important step forward in the future.

References

1. Lahuerta JJ, Mateos MV, Martinez-Lopez J et al. Busulfan 12 mg/kg plus melphalan 140 mg/m^2 versus melphalan 200 mg/m^2 as conditioning regimens for autologous transplantation in newly diagnosed multiple myeloma patients included in the PETHEMA/GEM2000 study. *Haematologica* 2010;95:1913–20.

2. Moreau P, Facon T, Attal M et al. Comparison of 200 mg/m^2 melphalan and 8 Gy total body irradiation plus 140 mg/m^2 melphalan as conditioning regimens for peripheral blood stem cell transplantation in patients with newly diagnosed multiple myeloma: final analysis of the Intergroupe Francophone du Myelome 9502 randomized trial. *Blood* 2002;99:731–5.

3. Lonial S, Kaufman J, Tighiouart M et al. A phase I/II trial combining high-dose melphalan and autologous transplant with bortezomib for multiple myeloma: a dose- and schedule-finding study. *Clin Cancer Res* 2010;16:5079–86.

4. Roussel M, Moreau P, Huynh A et al. Bortezomib and high-dose melphalan as conditioning regimen before autologous stem cell transplantation in patients with de novo multiple myeloma: a phase 2 study of the Intergroupe Francophone du Myelome (IFM). *Blood* 2010;115:32–7.

5. Sharma M, Zhang MJ, Zhong X et al. Older Patients with myeloma derive similar benefit from autologous transplantation. *Biol Blood Marrow Transplant* 2014;20:1796–803.

6. Badros A, Barlogie B, Siegel E et al. Results of autologous stem cell transplant in multiple myeloma patients with renal failure. *Br J Haematol* 2001;114:822–9.

7. Krishnan A, Pasquini MC, Logan B et al. Autologous haemopoietic stem-cell transplantation followed by allogeneic or autologous haemopoietic stem-cell transplantation in patients with multiple myeloma (BMT CTN 0102): a phase 3 biological assignment trial. *Lancet Oncol* 2011;12:1195–203.

8. Garban F, Attal M, Michallet M et al. Prospective comparison of autologous stem cell transplantation followed by dose-reduced allograft (IFM99-03 trial) with tandem autologous stem cell transplantation (IFM99-04 trial) in high-risk de novo multiple myeloma. *Blood* 2006;107:3474–80.

9. Kroger N, Perez-Simon JA, Myint H et al. Relapse to prior autograft and chronic graft-versus-host disease are the strongest prognostic factors for outcome of melphalan/fludarabine-based dose-reduced allogeneic stem cell transplantation in patients with multiple myeloma. *Biol Blood Marrow Transplant* 2004;10:698–708.

10. Caballero-Velazquez T, Lopez-Corral L, Encinas C et al. Phase II clinical trial for the evaluation of bortezomib within the reduced intensity conditioning regimen (RIC) and post-allogeneic transplantation for high-risk myeloma patients. *Br J Haematol* 2013;162:474–82.

11. Freytes CO, Vesole DH, Lerademacher J et al. Second transplants for multiple myeloma relapsing after a previous autotransplant-reduced-intensity allogeneic vs autologous transplantation. *Biol Bone Marrow Transplant* 2014;49:416–21.

12. Koreth J, Stevenson KE, Kim HT et al. Bortezomib-based graft-versus-host disease prophylaxis in HLA-mismatched unrelated donor transplantation. *J Clin Oncol* 2012;30:3202–8.

13. Garg TK, Szmania SM, Khan JA et al. Highly activated and expanded natural killer cells for multiple myeloma immunotherapy. *Haematologica* 2012;97:1348–56.

14. Kanold J, Paillard C, Tchirkov A et al. NK cell immunotherapy for high-risk neuroblastoma relapse after haploidentical HSCT. *Pediatr Blood Cancer* 2012;59:739–42.

15. Koehl U, Esser R, Zimmermann S et al. Ex vivo expansion of highly purified NK cells for immunotherapy after haploidentical stem cell transplantation in children. *Klin Padiatr* 2005;217:345–50.

16. Benson DM, Jr., Bakan CE, Zhang S et al. IPH2101, a novel anti-inhibitory KIR antibody, and lenalidomide combine to enhance the natural killer cell versus multiple myeloma effect. *Blood* 2011;118:6387–91.

17. Benson DM, Jr., Hofmeister CC, Padmanabhan S et al. A phase 1 trial of the anti-KIR antibody IPH2101 in patients with relapsed/refractory multiple myeloma. *Blood* 2012;120:4324–33.

8 Relapsed and refractory multiple myeloma

The choice of treatment for each stage of multiple myeloma (MM) involves a complex decision-making process, largely because of our growing understanding of plasma cell biology and the increase in therapeutic options at each stage of treatment. In addition to the established treatments (immunomodulatory drugs [IMiDs] and proteasome inhibitors), a number of new therapies have emerged, including second-generation proteasome inhibitors, histone deacetylase (HDAC) inhibitors (e.g. vorinostat and panobinostat) and monoclonal antibodies (Table 8.1). The treatment of relapsed or refractory multiple myeloma (RRMM) presents a special therapeutic challenge, because of the heterogeneity of disease at relapse and the absence of

TABLE 8.1
Current and emerging strategies for relapsed and refractory multiple myeloma

Current therapies	Emerging therapies
Immunomodulators	*Histone deacetylase inhibitors*
• Thalidomide	• Vorinostat
• Lenalidomide	• Panobinostat
• Pomalidomide	
	Proteasome inhibitors
Proteasome inhibitors	• Ixazomib
• Bortezomib	• Oprozomib
• Carfilzomib	
	Monoclonal antibodies
	• Elotuzumab
	• Daratumumab
	• Isatuximab
	• Pembrolizumab

clear biological-based recommendations regarding the choice of therapy at each stage of disease.

Definitions
According to the International Myeloma Working Group (IMWG) criteria, progressive disease is defined by one of the following:
- at least a 25% increase from nadir in serum or urine M protein levels (absolute increase must be ≥ 0.5 g/dL or ≥ 200 mg/24 hours, respectively)
- an abnormal serum free light chain (sFLC) ratio and normal/abnormal FLC difference greater than 100 mg/L.

In patients in whom M protein is not measurable, an increase in bone marrow plasma cells (≥ 10% increase), new bone or soft tissue lesions, increasing size of existing lesions or unexplained hypercalcemia (serum calcium > 11.5 mg/dL) is used to define disease progression.

'Relapsed and refractory' myeloma is defined as disease that has progressed on therapy in patients who achieve a minor response or better, or whose disease progresses within 60 days of their last therapy. Absence of at least a minor response to initial induction therapy and progression while on therapy is defined as 'primary refractory' MM. MM is defined as 'refractory' when it has previously been treated, there is evidence of progressive disease, as defined above, and, at the time of relapse, the criteria for 'relapsed and refractory' or 'primary refractory' myeloma are not met.

Historically, the duration of remission has decreased with each line of treatment, as the M protein load gradually increases. Recent European data indicate that this is still the case. However, as use of the monoclonal antibodies increases, longer periods of remission following relapse may become possible.

Factors influencing choice of treatment
The choice of treatment in patients with RRMM requires a balance between efficacy and toxicity. Factors to consider include:
- disease-related factors such as genetic risk

- treatment-related factors such as:
  - prior drug therapy
  - regimen-related toxicity (e.g. peripheral neuropathy and myelosuppression)
  - the depth and duration of response to previous drug treatment
- patient-related factors such as bone marrow function, renal and hepatic impairment, pre-existing neuropathy, comorbidities and performance status.

Immunomodulatory drugs

Thalidomide is the prototype IMiD used in myeloma but use is limited by the considerable neurotoxicity associated with long-term use. The addition of dexamethasone to thalidomide increases the objective response rate in patients with RRMM from about 24% to about 55%, and thalidomide is well tolerated in patients with renal failure and can be combined with proteasome inhibitors such as bortezomib and carfilzomib. In addition, thalidomide is not myelosuppressive, and thus may have a role in regimens containing dexamethasone with cyclophosphamide or melphalan for patients presenting with severe cytopenias. In patients with refractory myeloma, thalidomide can be combined with other agents such as vorinostat (see page 91), bortezomib or carfilzomib, achieving an overall clinical benefit rate above 70%, even in high-risk patients.

Lenalidomide is an analog of thalidomide that is more potent and has different toxicity. It was approved on the basis of two parallel trials that evaluated the addition of lenalidomide to dexamethasone in patients with RRMM who had received a median of two previous therapies. At a median follow-up of 48 months, patients receiving the combination showed a continuing benefit in terms of overall survival, although 47.6% of patients in the dexamethasone arm subsequently received lenalidomide-based treatment after disease progression or unblinding, which may have confounded the OS rate.

Clinical trials with lenalidomide-based combinations are summarized in Table 8.2. In general, combinations of lenalidomide with cytotoxic agents, monoclonal antibodies or proteasome inhibitors have achieved objective response rates of 65–95%, and higher-quality responses than comparator regimens. Chronic lenalidomide-induced diarrhea may be related to bile acid malabsorption and may respond to reduction in dietary fat intake, treatment with bile acid sequestrants, or both.

Pomalidomide is a third-generation IMiD; like the other agents in this class, it is significantly more active when combined with dexamethasone. The pomalidomide–dexamethasone combination was found to be strongly synergistic in both lenalidomide-sensitive and lenalidomide-resistant cell lines, inhibiting cell proliferation and inducing apoptosis. Clinical trials with pomalidomide in RRMM are summarized in Table 8.3. The combination of pomalidomide with dexamethasone has been evaluated in several Phase II trials and a large randomized Phase III trial, producing a response in approximately 30% of patients with lenalidomide-resistant MM, with a duration of 7–8 months. Pomalidomide can also be combined with carfilzomib and cyclophosphamide in a triplet, resulting in deeper responses in patients with RRMM (see Table 8.3). Evidence suggests that pomalidomide may be more effective in patients with del(17p) than in patients with the t(4;14) translocation; pomalidomide is therefore the first agent to demonstrate increased activity in del(17p) MM. This requires further investigation in order to incorporate pomalidomide into treatment strategies for this high-risk population.

Proteasome inhibitors
Bortezomib was the first proteasome inhibitor. Combinations with lenalidomide or thalidomide, alkylating agents (e.g. cyclophosphamide, bendamustine or melphalan), anthracyclines or HDAC inhibitors resulted in higher objective response rates (55–87%) than with bortezomib alone in trials, and can be considered in the management of RRMM. Trials with bortezomib in RRMM are summarized in Table 8.4. Re-treatment with bortezomib is feasible in selected patients with more than a partial response and remission lasting more than 6 months, provided that peripheral neuropathy is not present.

TABLE 8.2

Lenalidomide-based regimens used in the treatment of relapsed and refractory multiple myeloma

Study	N	Regimen
Richardson 2009[1] Phase II	222	R: R, 30 mg on days 1–21 every 28 days
Weber 2007[2] Phase III	177	RD: R, 25 mg/d on days 1–21; D, 40 mg/d on days 1–4, 9–12 and 17–20, orally every 28 days
	176	D: D, 40 mg/d on days 1–4, 9–12 and 17–20, orally every 28 days
Dimopoulos 2007[3] Phase III	176	RD: R, 25 mg/d on days 1–21; D, 40 mg/d on days 1–4, 9–12 and 17–20, orally every 28 days
	175	D: D, 40 mg/d on days 1–4, 9–12 and 17–20, orally every 28 days
Richardson 2012[4] Phase II	36	Rd+elotuzumab: E, 10 mg/kg iv qw x 2 cycles; q2w afterwards; R, 25 mg/d on days 1–21; D, 40 mg/d on days 1, 8, 15 and 22, orally every 28 days
	37	Rd+elotuzumab: E, 20 mg/kg iv qw x 2 cycles; q2w afterwards; R, 25 mg/d on days 1–21; D, 40 mg/d on days 1, 8, 15 and 22, orally every 28 days
Wang 2013[5] Phase II	52	CRd: C, 20/27 mg/m^2 on days 1, 2, 8, 9, 15, 16; R, 25 mg on days 1–21; D, 40 mg on days 1, 8, 15 and 22, every 28 days
Richardson 2014[6] Phase II	64	RVD: R, 15 mg/d on days 1–14; V, 1 mg/m^2 on days 1, 4, 8 and 11; D, 40/20 mg/d
Reece 2014[7] Phase I/II	32	CyPR: Cy, 300 mg/m^2 on days 1, 8 and 15; P, 100 mg qod; R, 25 mg on days 1–21, every 28 days

CRd, carfilzomib–lenalidomide–dexamethasone; CyPR, cyclophosphamide–prednisone–lenalidomide; d/D, low/high-dose dexamethasone; E, elotuzumab; P, prednisone; R: lenalidomide; Rd: lenalidomide–low-dose dexamethasone; RD: lenalidomide–high-dose dexamethasone; RVD, lenalidomide–bortezomib–dexamethasone.

Prior lines	≥ PR (%)	≥ VGPR (%)	PFS (mo)	OS (mo)
3	26		4.9	23.2
≥ 2	61	24.3	11.1	29.6
≥ 2	19.9 ($p < 0.001$)	1.7	4.7 ($p < 0.0001$)	20.2 ($p < 0.0001$)
≥ 2	60.2	24.4	11.3	NR
≥ 2	24 ($p < 0.0001$)	5.1	4.7 ($p < 0.0001$)	20.6 ($p = 0.03$)
≥ 2	92	61	26.9	NR
≥ 2	76	46	18.6	NR
NR	78	22	15.4	NR
2	64	28	9.5	30
2	94		16.1	27.6

iv, intravenous; mo, months; NR, not reported; OS, overall survival; PFS, progression-free survival; PR: partial response; qod: every other day; qw, every week; q2w, every 2 weeks; VGPR, very good partial response.

TABLE 8.3

Pomalidomide-based regimens used in the treatment of relapsed and refractory multiple myeloma

Study	N	Regimen
Lacy 2009[8] Phase II	60	Pd: P, 2 mg/d on days 1–21 every 28 days; D, 40 mg PO weekly
Richardson 2014[9] Phase II	113	Pd: P, 4 mg/d on days 1–21 every 28 days; D, 40 mg PO weekly
	108	P: P, 4 mg/d on days 1–21 every 28 days
San Miguel 2013[10] Phase III	302	Pd: P, 4 mg/d on days 1–21; D, 40 mg/d on days 1, 8, 15 and 22, PO
	153	D: D, 40 mg/d on days 1–4, 9–12 and 17–20, PO
Richardson 2013[11] Phase II	28	PVD: Dose escalation of P, from 1–4 mg/d; V, from 1–1.3 mg/m2; and D, 20 mg/d on days 1, 2, 4, 5, 8, 9, 11 and 12 every 28 days
Shah 2013[12] Phase I/II	72	CPd: CFZ, 20/27 mg/m² iv on days 1, 2, 8, 9, 15 and 16; P, 4 mg on days 1–21; D, 40 mg on days 1, 8, 15 and 22 every 28 days
Larocca 2013[13] Phase II	55	PdCyPr: P, 2.5 mg/d; Cy, 50 mg qod; and Pr, 50 mg qod every 28 days

CFZ, carfilzomib; CPd, carfilzomib–pomalidomide–dexamethasone;
Cy, cyclophosphamide; D: dexamethasone; P, pomalidomide;
Pd, pomalidomide–low-dose dexamethasone;
PdCyPr, pomalidomide–cyclophosphamide–prednisone;
Pr, prednisone; PVD, pomalidomide–bortezomib–dexamethasone.

Prior lines	≥ PR (%)	≥ VGPR (%)	PFS (mo)	OS (mo)
2	63	33	11.6	NR
5	33	NR	4.2	16.5
5	18 ($p = 0.013$)	NR	2.7 ($p = 0.003$)	13.6 ($p = 0.709$)
5	31	6	4	12.7
5	10 ($p < 0.001$)	< 1	1.9 ($p < 0.0001$)	8.1 ($p = 0.285$)
2	70	43	NR	NR
6	64	26.3	12	16.3
3	51	24	10.4	NR

iv, intravenous; mo, months; NR, not reported; OS, overall survival; PFS, progression-free survival; PO, per os; PR, partial response; qod, every other day; VGPR, very good partial response.

TABLE 8.4

Bortezomib-based regimens used in the treatment of relapsed and refractory multiple myeloma

Study	N	Regimen
Richardson 2003[14] Phase II	202	V: V, 1.3 mg/m² on days 1, 4, 8, 11 every 28 days
Richardson 2005[15] Phase III	333	V: V, 1.3 mg/m² on days 1, 4, 8, 11 every 21 days
	336	D: D, 40 mg on days 1–4, 9–12, 17–20 every 35 days
Orlowski 2007[16] Phase III	324	V-PLD: V, 1.3 mg/m² on days 1, 4, 8, 11 every 21 days; PLD, 30 mg/m² on day 4
	322	V: V, 1.3 mg/m² on days 1, 4, 8, 11 every 21 days
Garderet 2012[17] Phase III	135	VTD: V, 1.3 mg/m² on days 1, 4, 8, 11 every 21 days; T, 200 mg daily; D, 40 mg weekly
	134	TD: T, 200 mg daily; D, 40 mg weekly
Dimopoulos 2013[18] Phase III	317	V+vorinostat: V, 1.3 mg/m² on days 1, 4, 8, 11 every 21 days
	320	V: V, 1.3 mg/m² on days 1, 4, 8,11 every 21 days
Richardson 2013[19] Phase II	55	VD+panobinostat: V, 1.3 mg/m² on days 1, 4, 8, 11 every 21 days; panobinostat, 20 mg PO t.i.w.
Reece 2014[20] Phase I	98	VCyPr: V, 1.5 mg/m2 weekly; Cy, 300 mg/m²; Pr, 100 mg PO qod
San Miguel 2014[21] Phase III	387	VD+panobinostat: V, 1.3 mg/m² iv, on days 1, 4, 8, 11; D, 20 mg PO, on days 1, 2, 4, 5, 8, 9, 11, 12; panobinostat, 20 mg PO, on days 1, 3, 8, 10,12 every 21 days
	381	VD: V and D as above

Cy, cyclophosphamide; D, dexamethasone; PLD, pegylated liposomal doxorubicin; Pr, prednisone; T, thalidomide; V, bortezomib.

Prior lines	≥ PR (%)	≥ VGPR (%)	PFS (mo)	OS (mo)
6	27	10	7	16
2	38	7	6.2	29.8
2	18 ($p < 0.001$)	1 ($p < 0.001$)	3.5 ($p < 0.001$)	23.7 ($p = 0.0027$)
≥ 2	44	27	9.3	76% (15 mo)
≥ 2	41 ($p = 0.43$)	19 ($p = 0.015$)	6.5 ($p = 0.000004$)	65% (15 mo) ($p = 0.03$)
	87	56	18.3	71%
	72 ($p < 0.001$)	35 ($p < 0.001$)	13.6 ($p = 0.001$)	65% ($p = 0.09$)
2	56.2		7.63	NR
2	40 ($p < 0.001$)		6.83 ($p = 0.01$)	28.07 ($p = 0.0027$)
4	34.5		5.4	
2	68	42	15% (1yr)	89% (1y)
1–3	27.6*		11.99	33.64
1–3	15.7* ($p = 0.00006$)		8.08 ($p < 0.0001$)	30.39 ($p = 0.26$)

*Complete or near complete response; mo, months; OS, overall survival; PFS, progression-free survival; PO, per os; PR, partial response; qod, every other day; t.i.w., three times a week; VGPR, very good partial response; y, year.

Carfilzomib is an irreversible proteasome inhibitor that offers a number of advantages over bortezomib (a reversible inhibitor): more potent proteasome inhibition, efficacy in bortezomib-refractory patients and a significantly lower incidence of peripheral neuropathy. Clinical trials with this agent in RRMM are summarized in Table 8.5. The combination of carfilzomib and dexamethasone has shown good response rates, even in bortezomib-refractory patients. Similarly, combination therapy with carfilzomib, lenalidomide and

TABLE 8.5

Carfilzomib-based regimens used in the treatment of relapsed and refractory multiple myeloma

Study	N	Regimen
Siegel 2012[22] Phase II	266	CFZ: CFZ, 20 mg/m² iv on days 1, 2, 8, 9, 15 and 16 every 28 days in cycle 1, then 27 mg/m²
Vij 2012[23] Phase II	59	CFZ: CFZ, 20 mg/m² iv on days 1, 2, 8, 9, 15 and 16 every 28 days
	70	CFZ: CFZ, 20 mg/m² iv on days 1, 2, 8, 9, 15 and 16 every 28 days in cycle 1, then 27 mg/m²
Lendvai 2014[24] Phase II	42	CFZ: CFZ, 20 mg/m² iv on days 1, 2, 8, 9, 15 and 16 every 28 days in cycle 1, then 56 mg/m
Shah 2012[25] Phase I	20	CFZ+ARRY-520: CFZ, 20 mg/m² iv on days 1, 2, 8, 9, 15 and 16 every 28 days in cycle 1, then 29 mg/m²; ARRY-520 escalated from 0.75 mg/m² to 1.5 mg/m²
Kaufman 2013[26] Phase I	10	CFZ+panobinostat: CFZ, 20 mg/m² iv on days 1, 2, 8, 9, 15 and 16 every 28 days in cycle 1, then escalation to 36 mg/m²; panobinostat, 20 mg PO three times per week

CFZ, carfilzomib; iv, intravenous; mo, months; NR, not reported; OS, overall survival; PFS, progression free survival; PO, per os; PR, partial response; VGPR, very good partial response.

dexamethasone (CRD) results in high-quality responses in patients with RRMM. Favorable results were also obtained with carfilzomib in combination with pomalidomide and dexamethasone (CPD) in heavily pretreated patients who had received a median of six prior lines of therapy. A large Phase III trial in patients with relapsed myeloma who had received a median of two prior lines of therapy showed that CRD resulted in a significant improvement in progression-free survival (PFS).

Prior lines	≥ PR (%)	≥ VGPR (%)	PFS (mo)	OS (mo)
5	23.7	NR	3.7	15.6
2	42.4	17	8.2	NR
2	52.2	28.4	NR	NR
5	51	NR	4.1	20.3
4	35	5	NR	NR
NR	30	10	NR	NR

A disadvantage of carfilzomib is the need for consecutive days of administration, requiring six visits in a 28-day cycle. The ENDEAVOR study is currently evaluating a twice-weekly schedule of carfilzomib at higher doses (target dose of 56 mg/m^2).

Emerging therapies
Proteasome inhibitors
Ixazomib is a reversible proteasome inhibitor, currently in Phase III development. It is pharmacokinetically and pharmacodynamically distinct from bortezomib, with superior tissue penetration and greater biological activity. Weekly and twice-weekly dosage schedules have been evaluated in patients with RRMM, and preliminary data suggest that weekly dosing is effective and associated with less toxicity than twice-weekly dosing. Ixazomib is well tolerated, with low rates of peripheral neuropathy. In combination with lenalidomide and dexamethasone, twice-weekly ixazomib was well tolerated and resulted in greater depth of response than lenalidomide and dexamethasone alone. These results provide encouraging support for the possibility of a highly efficacious oral triplet induction regimen for patients with newly diagnosed or relapsed MM.

Oprozomib is an orally active derivative of carfilzomib. Preliminary data indicate promising activity as monotherapy in RRMM, and Phase I/II trials are continuing.

Histone deacetylase inhibitors
HDAC inhibitors prevent deacetylation of histone proteins, a process involved in the epigenetic regulation of gene expression that promotes cell proliferation and cell death. In myeloma cells, HDAC inhibitors inhibit cell growth and induce apoptosis when used as single agents, and are also synergistic with bortezomib. The clinical activity of HDAC inhibitors as single agents is limited but use in combination with dexamethasone or bortezomib in patients with RRMM overcomes bortezomib resistance. This is probably because of simultaneous inhibition of both protein handling pathways in the cell: the proteasome (bortezomib) and the aggresome/autophagy (HDAC inhibitor) systems. Several class-specific and pan-deacetylase inhibitors are currently in development.

Vorinostat. In a study evaluating vorinostat in combination with bortezomib in heavily pretreated patients with bortezomib-refractory disease, 17% achieved at least a partial response, and the clinical benefit rate was 31%. A further study in patients whose disease relapsed early showed a significant improvement in PFS with vorinostat plus bortezomib compared with bortezomib alone. The combination reduced the risk of progression by 23% compared with bortezomib alone, but the difference in PFS between the two groups was not clinically relevant. Although this combination offers a new therapeutic option for a difficult-to-treat patient population, overlapping toxicity is an issue: severe (grade 3 or above) thrombocytopenia occurred in 45% of patients receiving the combination, compared with 24% of those receiving bortezomib monotherapy.

Panobinostat. Preclinical studies demonstrated notable synergy between proteasome inhibitors and HDAC inhibitors in MM, which is related to the synergy that occurs when both the proteasome and aggresome pathways are blocked through combination therapy. Panobinostat, a novel hydroxamic acid-based pan-deacetylase inhibitor, has shown promising activity in combination with bortezomib in patients with RRMM.

In a Phase II study (PANORAMA 2), bortezomib, dexamethasone and panobinostat showed activity in heavily pretreated patients with bortezomib-refractory disease, with an objective response rate of 35% and clinical benefit rate of 53%. Median PFS was 5.5 months. This trial provided proof of principle that the addition of an HDAC inhibitor was able to overcome bortezomib resistance.

A large randomized Phase III trial (PANORAMA 1) that evaluated the addition of panobinostat to bortezomib and dexamethasone has further validated the efficacy of this combination, though not in all patients. The panobinostat combination produced a significant improvement in median PFS compared with bortezomib and dexamethasone (see Table 8.4). The benefit of the addition of panobinostat was most marked in patients who had been exposed to both bortezomib and lenalidomide and in patients with high-risk genetics. The most common grade 3/4 adverse events reported with the panobinostat combination compared with the doublet were diarrhea (25.5% versus 8.8%), thrombocytopenia (47.1% versus 5.9%) and fatigue (14.7% versus 2.0%).

Panobinostat has received accelerated approval from the US Food and Drug Administration on the basis of these results, for use in patients with RRMM.

More selective HDAC inhibitors are in development, and Phase I/II trials of combinations with proteasome inhibitors and IMiDs are ongoing. It is hoped that these will provide additional safety and efficacy data for this new and important class of agents.

Monoclonal antibodies

Elotuzumab is a humanized monoclonal antibody that targets the cell surface glycoprotein CS1 (also known as SLAMF7). Elotuzumab mediates antibody-dependent cell-mediated cytotoxicity (ADCC) in myeloma cell lines and myeloma cells from patients with MM that is resistant or refractory to conventional therapies and bortezomib. In a Phase I trial, objective responses were observed in 23 of 28 patients (82%) receiving a combination of elotuzumab with lenalidomide and dexamethasone. In a subsequent Phase II extension phase, response rates of up to 92% and median PFS of up to 33 months were reported in patients receiving elotuzumab, 10 or 20 mg/kg, with no dose-limiting toxicities.

The recently published results of the ELOQUENT 2 trial, which evaluated the addition of elotuzumab to lenalidomide plus low-dose dexamethasone (Rd) for patients with relapsed MM, include significantly improved objective response rate and PFS with the elotuzumab-containing regimen, and a trend towards improved OS.[27] The time to next therapy was also longer in the elotuzumab group, and data suggest that patients with high-risk disease also fared better with this regimen.

The ELOQUENT 1 study is a similarly designed phase III trial evaluating the addition of elotuzumab to lenalidomide plus low-dose dexamethasone in patients with newly diagnosed MM or relapsed MM; results are expected in a couple of years.

Daratumumab is a humanized anti-CD38 monoclonal antibody that directly targets tumor cells and also mediates the killing of CD38-expressing plasma cells via ADCC, antibody-dependent cellular phagocytosis (ADCP), complement-dependent cytotoxicity (CDC) and apoptosis. In a Phase I dose-escalation study in heavily pretreated patients, marked reductions in M protein and bone marrow plasma cells were observed at doses of 4 mg/kg and above, and 42% of patients achieved at least a partial response at these doses. In a large Phase II study in patients with refractory MM, the objective response rate with daratumumab monotherapy was 30% in more than 100 patients who had previously received a median of five prior lines of therapy.[28] Furthermore, in-vitro studies using ADCC assays showed that the combination of daratumumab and lenalidomide enhanced natural killer cell-mediated cytotoxicity.

Preliminary results from a Phase I/II study of daratumumab in combination with lenalidomide and oral dexamethasone in patients with RRMM suggest that the combination has a manageable safety profile consistent with that of lenalidomide, and an encouraging 75% objective response rate. Two large randomized phase III trials in the past 12 months have demonstrated the benefit of adding daratumumab to standard salvage regimens. The Castor trial demonstrated that the addition of daratumumab to bortezomib plus dexamethasone in patients with early relapse achieved a significant improvement in the objective response rate, complete response rate and PFS. A similarly designed study, the POLLUX trial, evaluated the addition of daratumumab to Rd, also showing significant improvements in objective response rate, PFS and minimal residual disease negativity. Median PFS has not yet been reached in the POLLUX trial and is estimated at 40 months – the longest PFS ever seen in a relapsed MM Phase III trial. These two trials have established the role of daratumumab in late and early relapse.

Isatuximab is another humanized anti-CD38 monoclonal antibody with strong pro-apoptotic activity; as with daratumumab, cytotoxicity is mediated by ADCC, ADCP and CDC. In a Phase I dose-escalation study in patients with selected CD38+ hematologic malignancies, the maximum tolerated dose of isatuximab was not reached with doses of up to 10 mg/kg once weekly, and the only dose-limiting toxicities were grade 2 infusion reactions. Among six patients with MM who received 10 mg/kg every 2 weeks, three had a partial response and two had stable disease.

Encouraging findings have also been reported for combinations of isatuximab with proteasome inhibitors and lenalidomide, supporting the notion that monoclonal antibodies can be safely combined with the two most active classes of anti-myeloma agents. As with elotuzumab and daratumumab, the combination of isatuximab with IMiDs appears to be particularly promising.

Pembrolizumab is a monoclonal antibody targeted at PD-1 (programmed cell death protein 1) that is approved for the treatment of lung cancer and melanoma. Pembrolizumab has no activity in MM as a single agent; however, in a Phase II trial that evaluated pembrolizumab in combination with Rd, the objective response rate was 50% for the trial population as a whole and 38% among patients who were resistant to Rd (more than half of the enrolled patients).

Key points – relapsed and refractory multiple myeloma

- Management of relapsed and refractory multiple myeloma (RRMM) continues to be challenging because of the clinical and genetic heterogeneity of patients.
- Currently available proteasome inhibitors and immunomodulatory drugs (IMiDs), used with dexamethasone or doublets, have improved response rates in this population, with some durable responses.
- Second-generation proteasome inhibitors and histone deacetylase (HDAC) inhibitors are promising agents in combination with currently available therapy.
- The most significant advance over the last 2 years has been the emergence of effective monoclonal antibodies directed against SLAM7 (elotuzumab) and CD38 (daratumumab, isatuximab). Objective response rates in combination with IMiDs in heavily pretreated patients are highly encouraging.

Ongoing Phase III studies are evaluating the combination of pembrolizumab with lenalidomide, as are studies testing the PD-1 inhibitor nivolumab, and the PD-L1 (programmed death-ligand 1) inhibitor durvalumab.

References

1. Richardson P, Jagannath S, Hussein M et al. Safety and efficacy of single-agent lenalidomide in patients with relapsed and refractory multiple myeloma. *Blood* 2009;114:772–8.

2. Weber DM, Chen C, Niesvizky R et al. Lenalidomide plus dexamethasone for relapsed multiple myeloma in North America. *N Engl J Med* 2007;357:2133–42.

3. Dimopoulos M, Spencer A, Attal M et al. Lenalidomide plus dexamethasone for relapsed or refractory multiple myeloma. *N Engl J Med* 2007;357:2123–32.

4. Richardson PG, Jagannath S, Moreau P et al. A phase 2 study of elotuzumab (Elo) in combination with lenalidomide and low-dose dexamethasone (Ld) in patients (pts) with relapsed/refractory multiple myeloma (R/R MM): Updated Results. *ASH Meeting Abstracts*, 16 November. 2012;120:202.

5. Wang M, Martin T, Bensinger W et al. Phase 2 dose-expansion study (PX-171-006) of carfilzomib, lenalidomide, and low-dose dexamethasone in relapsed or progressive multiple myeloma. *Blood* 2013;122:3122–8.

6. Richardson PG, Xie W, Jagannath S et al. A phase 2 trial of lenalidomide, bortezomib, and dexamethasone in patients with relapsed and relapsed/refractory myeloma. *Blood* 2014;123:1461–9.

7. Reece DE, Masih-Khan E, Atenafu EG et al. Phase I-II trial of oral cyclophosphamide, prednisone and lenalidomide for the treatment of patients with relapsed and refractory multiple myeloma. *Br J Haematol* 2015;168:46–54.

8. Lacy MQ, Hayman SR, Gertz MA et al. Pomalidomide (CC4047) plus low-dose dexamethasone as therapy for relapsed multiple myeloma. *J Clin Oncol* 2009;27:5008–14.

9. Richardson PG, Siegel DS, Vij R et al. Pomalidomide alone or in combination with low-dose dexamethasone in relapsed and refractory multiple myeloma: a randomized phase 2 study. *Blood* 2014;123:1826–32.

10. San Miguel J, Hungria VT, Yoon S-S et al. Efficacy and safety based on duration of treatment of panobinostat plus bortezomib and dexamethasone in patients with relapsed and refractory multiple myeloma in the Phase 3 Panorama 1 study. *Blood* 2014; 124:4742.

11. Richardson PG, Hofmeister CC, Siegel D et al. MM-005: A phase 1 trial of pomalidomide, bortezomib, and low-dose dexamethasone (PVD) in relapsed and/or refractory multiple myeloma (RRMM). *Blood* 2013;122:1969.

12. Shah JJ, Stadtmauer EA, Abonour R et al. Phase I/II dose expansion of a multi-center trial of carfilzomib and pomalidomide with dexamethasone (Car-Pom-d) in patients with relapsed/refractory multiple myeloma. *Blood* 2013;122:690.

13. Larocca A, Montefusco V et al. Pomalidomide, cyclophosphamide, and prednisone for relapsed/refractory multiple myeloma: a multicenter phase 1/2 open-label study. *Blood* 2013;122:2799–806.

14. Richardson PG, Barlogie B, Berenson J et al. A phase 2 study of bortezomib in relapsed, refractory myeloma. *N Engl J Med* 2003;348:2609–17.

15. Richardson PG, Sonneveld P, Schuster MW et al. Bortezomib or high-dose dexamethasone for relapsed multiple myeloma. *N Engl J Med* 2005;352:2487–98.

16. Orlowski RZ, Nagler A, Sonneveld P et al. Randomized phase III study of pegylated liposomal doxorubicin plus bortezomib compared with bortezomib alone in relapsed or refractory multiple myeloma: combination therapy improves time to progression. *J Clin Oncol* 2007;25:3892–901.

17. Garderet L, Iacobelli S, Moreau P et al. Superiority of the triple combination of bortezomib-thalidomide-dexamethasone over the dual combination of thalidomide-dexamethasone in patients with multiple myeloma progressing or relapsing after autologous transplantation. *J Clin Oncol* 2012;30:2475–82.

18. Dimopoulos M, Siegel DS, Lonial S et al. Vorinostat or placebo in combination with bortezomib in patients with multiple myeloma (VANTAGE 088): a multicentre, randomised, double-blind study. *Lancet Oncol* 2013;14:1129–40.

19. Richardson PG, Schlossman RL, Alsina M et al. PANORAMA 2: panobinostat in combination with bortezomib and dexamethasone in patients with relapsed and bortezomib-refractory myeloma. *Blood* 2013;122:2331–7.

20. Reece DE, Trieu Y, Masih-Khan E et al. Treatment of relapsed/refractory multiple myeloma with weekly cyclophosphamide plus bortezomib plus prednisone or dexamethasone (CyBor-P/D): Updated experience at Princess Margaret Cancer Centre (PMCC). *ASCO Meeting Abstracts*, June 11. 2014;32(15suppl):e19568.

21. San Miguel J, Weisel K, Moreau P et al. Pomalidomide plus low-dose dexamethasone versus high-dose dexamethasone alone for patients with relapsed and refractory multiple myeloma (MM-003): a randomised, open-label, phase 3 trial. *Lancet Oncol* 2013;14:1055–66.

22. Siegel DS, Martin T, Wang M et al. A phase 2 study of single-agent carfilzomib (PX-171-003-A1) in patients with relapsed and refractory multiple myeloma. *Blood* 2012;120:2817–25.

23. Vij R, Siegel DS, Jagannath S et al. An open-label, single-arm, phase 2 study of single-agent carfilzomib in patients with relapsed and/or refractory multiple myeloma who have been previously treated with bortezomib. *Br J Haematol* 2012;158:739–48.

24. Lendvai N, Hilden P, Devlin S et al. A phase 2 single-center study of carfilzomib 56 mg/m^2 with or without low-dose dexamethasone in relapsed multiple myeloma. *Blood* 2014;124:899–906.

25. Shah JJ, Weber DM, Thomas SK et al. Phase 1 Study of the novel kinesin spindle protein inhibitor ARRY-520 + carfilzomib in patients with relapsed and/or refractory multiple myeloma. *Blood* 2012;12:4082.

26. Kaufman J, Zimmerman T, Jakubowiak A et al. Phase I study of combination of carfilzomib and panabinostat for patients with relapsed and refractory myeloma: a multicenter MMRC clinical trial. *18th Congress of European Hematology Association*, 13–16 June 2013; Stockholm, Sweden.

27. Lonial S, Dimopoulos M, Palumbo A et al. Elotuzumab therapy for relapsed or refractory multiple myeloma. *New Engl J Med* 2015;373:621–31.

28. Lonial S, Weiss BM, Usmani SZ et al. Daratumumab monotherapy in patients with treatment-refractory multiple myeloma (SIRIUS): an open-label, randomised, phase 2 trial. *Lancet* 2016;387(10027):1551–60.

9 Bone disease and renal complications

Bone disease

Osteolytic bone damage is a key feature of multiple myeloma (MM), and bone pain and fracture of the ribs, long bones or vertebrae are often the initial presenting symptoms (Table 9.1); up to 80% of patients have bone lesions on skeletal radiography at diagnosis. Patients frequently have concomitant symptomatic hypercalcemia, spinal cord compression or both, which can lead to emergency hospital admissions. Myeloma-related bone disease appears to be a key contributory factor to poor performance status: limited mobility secondary to fractures and bone pain leads to reduced exercise tolerance, decreased muscle mass, frequent chest infections, fatigue and loss of economic activity in patients of working age.

Clinical presentation. Bone resorption, and subsequent bone destruction manifesting as lytic lesions and fractures, is a characteristic feature of MM (Figure 9.1), distinguishing MM from all other malignancies. Common presenting features include back pain, pain in the ribs or fracture of a long bone, which often prompt visits to a primary care practitioner or emergency department. Often, patients are managed with painkillers and investigated with skeletal

TABLE 9.1

Signs and symptoms of myeloma-related bone disease

- Back pain
- Bone pain
- Fractures of the long bones, ribs or both
- Vertebral fractures
- Symptomatic hypercalcemia
- Spinal cord compression
- Bone lesions on skeletal radiography

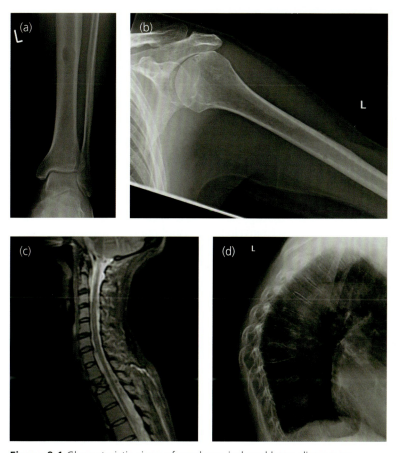

Figure 9.1 Characteristic signs of myeloma-induced bone disease on skeletal radiography: (a) tibial lytic lesion; (b) humeral lytic lesions; (c) vertebral compression fractures with marrow infiltration; (d) vertebral compression fractures.

radiography (see pages 41–42), which can miss early myeloma bone lesions. Not infrequently, however, pain can be more severe and patients may be admitted to hospital – usually under orthopedic teams – with bone pain, fractures or neurological complications resulting from fractures. Significant osteopenia, and occasionally osteoporosis without fractures, have also been described in patients with MM.

Although not all patients with MM present with overt bone disease, bone lesions can potentially develop during the course of the disease.

In a population-based retrospective cohort study, 16 times more fractures were observed than would have been expected in the year before the diagnosis of MM, mostly pathological fractures of the vertebrae and ribs. Patients often continue to experience bone pain and progressive skeletal morbidity after initial surgical or conservative management of fractures; this pain can significantly limit mobility and reduce quality of life. Vertebral lesions in patients with MM lead to loss of height, exaggerated kyphosis (forward curvature of the spine), reduced respiratory reserve and frequent chest infections.

Pathophysiology. Myeloma bone disease occurs as a result of the interaction between myeloma cells and the bone marrow microenvironment. Crucially, this interaction is also necessary for myeloma cell growth and survival (as described in Chapter 2), and the ensuing vicious cycle serves to enhance the destructive nature of myeloma bone disease.

Uncoupling of osteoblast and osteoclast activity in the bones of patients with MM is primarily due to osteoclast activation and inhibition of osteoblast maturation and function. Osteoclasts are activated by a number of cytokines, including the receptor activator of nuclear factor (NF)-κB (RANK) ligand (RANKL), which induces differentiation, formation, fusion and survival of pre-osteoclasts, as well as directly activating mature osteoclasts. In addition, osteoblastic lineage cells and stromal cells secrete osteoprogerin (OPG), a decoy receptor antagonist for RANKL: a balanced RANKL/OPG ratio is essential for normal bone turnover, and an imbalance in this ratio in the tumor microenvironment is central to the development of osteolytic disease. Suppression of osteoblastogenesis in MM through inhibition of the Wnt pathway and other signaling pathways leads to decreased OPG formation, resulting in an abnormal RANKL/OPG ratio and decreased bone production. Myeloma-induced bone disease is likely to be ameliorated by suppression of osteoclast formation and enhancement of osteoblast activity, in parallel with inducing remission.

Imaging. Skeletal radiography is the standard screening technique at diagnosis for all patients with MM, and can detect lytic lesions, osteopenia and fractures. However, lesions are not visualized on radiography until up to 30% of cancellous bone has been lost. MRI of the whole spine and pelvis should therefore be considered in all patients with MM, to provide additional information to guide clinical management.

MRI of the spine is the procedure of choice for identification of edema in acute vertebral fractures and associated soft tissue, with detailed neurological evaluation. CT scanning of the spine is useful to assess spinal stability in patients with vertebral fractures. Whole-body MRI and PET-CT are more sensitive than skeletal radiography in identifying myeloma-related bone disease in the axial and appendicular skeleton, and to accurately stage patients with monoclonal gammopathy of undetermined significance (MGUS) and asymptomatic myeloma.[1]

Biochemical markers of bone disease. Measurement of bone turnover markers in patients with MM is complicated by large random intra-patient variability, biological variability and poor standardization of most assays, which have confounded widespread use of these assays in clinical practice. Potential bone turnover markers are shown in Table 9.2.

Clinically, urinary NTX, serum CTX, serum P1NP and BALP are useful measures of bone remodeling in MM, and these markers can be used to optimize bisphosphonate use in the management of bone disease in patients with MM.

TABLE 9.2
Biochemical markers of bone formation and resorption

Bone formation	Bone resorption
• Bone-specific alkaline phosphatase (BALP)	• N-telopeptide of type 1 collagen (NTX)
• Osteocalcin	• C-terminal telopeptide of type 1 collagen (CTX)
• N-terminal propeptide of type 1 procollagen (P1NP)	• Pyridinoline cross-links

Treatment and prevention. Lifestyle optimization and general measures can have a significant effect in managing bone disease.
- Weight reduction, smoking cessation, adequate calcium intake and regular exercise have been shown to optimize bone health in patients with osteoporosis, and are applicable to patients with MM.
- Patients with MM are often vitamin D deficient, and vitamin D supplementation is crucial before starting bisphosphonate therapy to ensure good absorption of dietary calcium.
- Patients with vertebral bone disease will benefit from spinal stabilization to prevent progressive kyphosis and improve respiratory function.

Bisphosphonates, which induce osteoclast apoptosis, are the standard of care for myeloma-related bone disease. In the clinical setting, treatment with pamidronate or zoledronic acid significantly reduces pain related to bone disease and prevents skeletal-related events. Zoledronic acid also appears to provide a survival advantage compared with oral sodium clodronate. However, there is no role for bisphosphonates in patients with MGUS or smoldering myeloma.

Adverse effects of bisphosphonate therapy include infusion reactions, renal impairment, atypical bone fractures and osteonecrosis of the jaw. The last can be prevented by maintaining good dental hygiene and temporary interruption of bisphosphonates. Invasive dental procedures should be avoided when possible, and dental health should be monitored annually; temporary discontinuation of bisphosphonates should be considered if invasive dental procedures are necessary. Renal function should be monitored monthly and patients should receive calcium and vitamin D supplements.[2]

Denosumab is a humanized monoclonal antibody (mAb) that targets the RANK ligand, administered subcutaneously. It is approved by the US Food and Drug Administration for the treatment of osteoporosis and the prevention of skeletal-related events in patients with solid tumors. A Phase III trial in patients with newly diagnosed MM showed denosumab to be non-inferior to zoledronic acid in preventing or delaying skeletal-related events.[3] This could change clinical practice for patients with MM, as denosumab can be delivered in the community setting and used in patients with poor renal function.

Low-dose radiation (up to 30 Gy) can be used as palliative treatment for uncontrolled pain and impending pathological fracture or spinal cord compression. Radiotherapy should be used judiciously, however, depending on the clinical presentation and the need for urgent response. The radiotherapy field should be limited in order to spare the patient's bone marrow function.

Multidisciplinary approach. The management of myeloma-related spinal disease requires a multidisciplinary approach comprising:
- treatment of the myeloma with systemic chemotherapy
- adequate pain control
- relief of cord or cauda equina compression and measures to reduce the risk of further bony destruction that can lead to spinal deformity or neurological dysfunction.

Drug treatment (anti-myeloma therapy, bisphosphonates, opiate analgesics), radiotherapy or both may not adequately relieve pain in some patients. In this situation, spinal bracing may provide short-term pain control by stabilizing the spine and reducing the mechanical load on the vertebral bodies; surgical intervention should be reserved for significant spinal instability. Vertebral augmentation is indicated for significant pain affecting day-to day function resulting from vertebral compression fractures or bone destruction with high risk of collapse. Minimally invasive vertebral augmentation techniques, percutaneous vertebroplasty and balloon kyphoplasty have been shown to decrease pain associated with vertebral compression fractures.

Renal damage

Renal impairment is a common and potentially serious complication of MM. Up to 25% of patients have some degree of renal dysfunction at diagnosis, and up to 50% of patients experience renal impairment at some time during their disease. Renal insufficiency can be reversed in approximately 50% of patients, but a large proportion will have some degree of persistent renal impairment and 2–12% of these will require renal replacement therapy. Outcomes in patients with renal impairment are poor because of high early mortality rates. Patients with newly diagnosed MM and renal failure are usually excluded from clinical trials, and the lack of trials in these patients is a concern.

Pathophysiology. Common forms of kidney injury in patients with newly diagnosed MM with acute kidney disease and excessive monoclonal protein, include:
- cast nephropathy, in which casts of filtered monoclonal immunoglobulin (Ig) and other urinary proteins obstruct distal renal tubules, causing tubulointerstitial nephritis
- AL amyloidosis, in which amyloidogenic monoclonal light chains are deposited in the glomeruli
- monoclonal immunoglobulin deposition disease (MIDD), in which light or heavy chains are deposited along the glomerular membranes or tubular basement membranes.

M protein injures renal tissue in several ways. Light chains may precipitate or form casts, leading to proximal tubule dysfunction and interstitial inflammation in tubular epithelial cells. In addition, the processing of pathologically large quantities of light chains by proximal tubular cells may result in the production of proinflammatory cytokines and epithelial–mesenchymal transformation of tubular epithelial cells, which contributes to inflammatory cell infiltration, matrix deposition and fibrosis. MIDD is generally associated with kappa (κ) light chains, which may be fragmented or abnormally large and may have atypical glycosylation or amino acid patterns that lead to misfolding, insolubility and precipitation. By contrast, AL amyloidosis is usually associated with lambda (λ) light chains, which appear to induce a fibroblast phenotype in mesangial cells, resulting in matrix deposition.

Investigation. A kidney biopsy is often required to confirm the type of renal injury in both Ig-dependent and -independent renal impairment. Measurement of M protein by immunofixation in serum and urine is also helpful in diagnosis; analysis of free light chains (FLCs) in serum is useful in oliguric patients and can replace urine electrophoresis.

Acute medical management will correct modest renal impairment in a substantial proportion of patients. Intravascular volume should be restored to ensure a steady flow of urine in non-oliguric patients, avoiding the use of loop diuretics where possible. Alkalinization of the urine is of unproven benefit and risks increasing calcium and phosphate deposition in the kidneys and elsewhere, particularly if hypercalcemia or hyperphosphatemia are present.

Hypercalcemia should be treated with intravenous saline, diuretics and bisphosphonates at doses appropriate for patients with renal impairment. Rasburicase (recombinant urate oxidase) is effective in the treatment of hyperuricemia in patients with tumor lysis. Non-steroidal anti-inflammatory drugs (NSAIDs) and renin-angiotensin inhibitors must be avoided; N-acetyl cysteine prophylaxis should be used if injection of contrast medium is required for imaging.

Management of the plasma cell clone. Some 50% of patients with MM who have raised urinary FLC excretion have renal impairment, compared with only 2% of those who do not have urinary FLC excretion. High-dose dexamethasone should be started immediately in patients with MM and renal failure (unless contraindicated), pending initiation of definitive treatment. Plasma exchange is not beneficial in patients with newly diagnosed MM with renal impairment, and its value in monoclonal Ig-associated kidney injury remains uncertain: the high volume of distribution of light chains and IgG results in low clearance relative to body stores, and rapid plasma refill occurs after each apheresis session.

Bortezomib-based therapy is preferred because of the rapid responses seen. Evidence from the MERIT trial and retrospective studies indicate that lowering sFLC levels within weeks of diagnosis increases the likelihood of being alive and dialysis free at 100 days. Thus, an early treatment switch should be considered if sFLC levels have not decreased within the first 3 weeks of therapy; alkylating agents can be added once renal function improves. High cut-off dialysis during initial therapy does not appear to confer any significant increase in renal recovery.

Monoclonal gammopathy of renal significance (MGRS, described in Chapter 2, page 21) is diagnosed from characteristic findings on renal biopsy. Chemotherapy should be considered for patients with stages 1–3 chronic kidney disease (CKD), in order to slow progression to end-stage renal disease.[4] Bortezomib- or thalidomide-based regimens with low-dose cyclophosphamide are the best options; bendamustine can also be used. Autologous stem cell transplantation (ASCT) may be appropriate in selected responding patients, although the long-term benefit of this strategy in preserving renal function remains to be proven.

For patients with stage 4–5 CKD who are eligible for renal transplantation, chemotherapy with ASCT should be considered either before or after transplantation. However, chemotherapy confers minimal benefit in patients who are not candidates for renal transplantation.

Key points – bone disease and renal complications

- Up to 80% of patients have bone lesions on skeletal radiography at diagnosis.
- Patients with bone disease should receive regular bisphosphonate therapy.
- Treatment of myeloma-related spinal disease requires a multidisciplinary approach, including supportive measures.
- Cast nephropathy, monoclonal immunoglobulin deposition disease and AL amyloidosis are common causes of renal impairment in patients with plasma cell dyscrasias.
- Patients with monoclonal gammopathy of renal significance and chronic kidney disease require active treatment to prevent deterioration of renal function.
- Multiple myeloma (MM) with renal failure is an emergency, and treatment should be started as soon as possible.
- Supportive measures with steroids improve kidney function in the majority of patients with MM and renal failure.

References

1. Dimopoulos M, Terpos E, Comenzo RL et al. International myeloma working group consensus statement and guidelines regarding the current role of imaging techniques in the diagnosis and monitoring of multiple myeloma. *Leukemia* 2009;23:1545–56.

2. Terpos E, Morgan G, Dimopoulos MA et al. International Myeloma Working Group recommendations for the treatment of multiple myeloma-related bone disease. *J Clin Oncol* 2013;31:2347–57.

3. Terpos E, Raje N, Durie BG et al. Comparison of denosumab vs zoledronic acid for treatment of bone disease in adults with newly diagnosed multiple myeloma: a randomized, double-blind, multinational phase 3 trial. *Ann Oncol* 2014; 25 (suppl 4): iv540.

4. Fermand JP, Bridoux F, Kyle RA et al. How I treat monoclonal gammopathy of renal significance (MGRS). *Blood* 2013;122:3583–90.

10 AL amyloidosis

Amyloidosis is a rare but serious disease caused by accumulation of abnormal insoluble protein fibers, known as amyloid fibrils, in the extracellular space in the tissues. There are various forms of amyloid disease, which differ in terms of the protein precursor that aggregates and the target organs in which amyloid is deposited, reflected in their clinical presentation; these range from localized cerebral amyloidosis in neurodegenerative conditions to systemic amyloidosis. Several different causative precursor proteins have been identified, such as immunoglobulin (Ig) monoclonal light chain in amyloid light-chain (AL) amyloidosis and transthyretin (TTR) amyloidosis (ATTR) (Table 10.1).

Distinct therapeutic approaches are required for each type of amyloidosis, as they vary in clinical course and the organs that need to be targeted. It is therefore essential to definitively identify the protein responsible for the disease before counseling the patient and commencing therapy.

AL amyloidosis is the most common form of systemic amyloidosis. It is a rare, incurable disorder caused by the deposition of amyloid

TABLE 10.1

Types of amyloidosis and precursor protein and site of production

Type	Amyloidogenic protein
AL amyloidosis (reactive or hereditary)	Light chain or immunoglobulin
AA amyloidosis (reactive)	Serum amyloid A
Senile systemic amyloidosis (hereditary)	Transthyretin (wild type)
Transthyretin amyloidosis (hereditary)	Mutant transthyretin
Fibrinogen amyloidosis (hereditary)	Variant fibrinogen
Apolipoprotein amyloidosis (hereditary)	Variant apolipoprotein

Amyloidogenic protein is produced in the bone marrow in AL amyloidosis but in the liver in all other types.

fibrils derived from clonal proteins that usually originate from an underlying plasma cell dyscrasia, or occasionally from a low-grade B-cell lymphoproliferative disorder. It is a disorder of protein folding, characterized by extracellular accumulation of β-pleated fibrillar deposits of monoclonal Ig light-chain fragments, which eventually leads to organ dysfunction (Figure 10.1). The most commonly affected organs are the kidneys, heart, liver and peripheral nervous system (Figure 10.2).

The clinical presentation is highly variable because of differences in organ involvement and a poor correlation between the amount of amyloid and the degree of impairment, particularly in the kidneys.

Untreated progressive systemic AL amyloidosis leads to multiorgan failure, which is associated with poor performance status and is fatal in more than 50% of patients. However, treatments that reduce the supply of amyloidogenic monoclonal Ig light chains can stabilize the disease or cause regression of existing amyloid deposits, leading to preservation or improvement in organ function and improved survival.

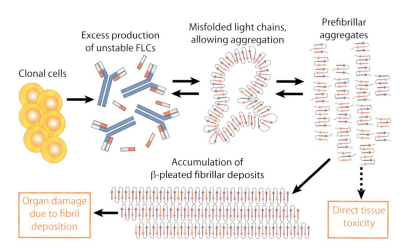

Figure 10.1 In AL amyloidosis, an abnormally proliferative monoclonal population of plasma cells produce immunoglobulin light chains. Once in the circulation, the proteins misfold into an insoluble β-pleated sheet configuration. Amyloid fibrils are deposited in numerous tissues and organs, causing organ failure and death. FLCs, free light chains.

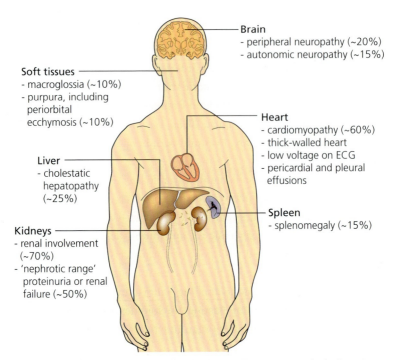

Figure 10.2 Patients with AL amyloidosis usually present with dysfunction of one or more organs, most typically renal involvement, cardiomyopathy, cholestatic hepatopathy, peripheral or autonomic neuropathy, or infiltration of soft tissues.

Epidemiology

The age-adjusted incidence of AL amyloidosis in the USA is 5.1–12.8 per million persons per year, and men and women are affected equally. In the UK, the incidence of AL amyloidosis is estimated at 0.8 per 100 000 population, and the disease accounts for about 1 in 1500 deaths. The incidence increases with age: in a study from the Mayo Clinic in the USA, 60% of patients were 50–70 years of age at diagnosis and only 10% were under 50 years.[1] Similarly, data from the UK indicate that 28% of patients were aged over 70 years at diagnosis, 62% were aged 50–70 years, 10% were under 50 years, and 2% were under 40 years. However, there may be a referral bias, as elderly patients with poor performance status are unlikely to be seen in centers of excellence.

Pathophysiology

AL amyloidosis often results from an underlying plasma cell dyscrasia classified as monoclonal gammopathy of undetermined significance (MGUS) because of low-level plasma cell infiltration. Although coexistent AL amyloidosis is diagnosed in 10–15% of patients who present with overt myeloma, the clinical presentation is not dominated by AL amyloid deposition. MGUS rarely progresses to overt myeloma in patients with AL amyloidosis, partly because of the inherently poor survival with the latter. AL amyloidosis can also complicate certain B-cell malignancies such as Waldenström's macroglobulinemia (lymphoplasmacytic lymphoma) and marginal zone lymphoma.

AL amyloid fibrils are derived from the N-terminal region of monoclonal Ig light chains and consist of the whole of the variable domain or, more commonly, just a part of it (see Figure 3.3, page 30). All monoclonal light chains are structurally unique and only a small proportion are amyloidogenic; however, lambda (λ) light chains are about three times more likely than kappa (κ) light chains to be associated with amyloid formation. The propensity for certain light chains to form amyloid fibrils is an inherent property related to their specific structure.

Genetic abnormalities, as noted in multiple myeloma (MM) plasma cell clones, have been observed in AL amyloidosis: the t(11;14) translocation is significantly more common in AL amyloidosis than in MM, whereas hyperdiploidy and the poor-risk MM t(4;14) and del(17p) genetic abnormalities are rare.

Clinical presentation

AL amyloidosis has an insidious onset and shows considerable heterogeneity in clinical presentation; a high level of clinical suspicion is therefore essential to make an early diagnosis. The disease can be either localized or systemic.

Localized disease involves only a single organ, frequently affecting the upper respiratory, urogenital or gastrointestinal tracts, the skin or the orbit. In this situation, the amyloidogenic light chains are produced by an inconspicuous focal infiltrate of clonal lymphoplasmacytoid cells within the same tissue as the amyloid deposits. Localized amyloidosis is often nodular but can also occur diffusely throughout a particular tissue. The AL nature of localized amyloid can often be confirmed immunohistochemically or by proteomic analysis, although it may not be possible to characterize the associated clonal cells because of the low level of infiltration. Monoclonal Ig cannot be detected in the serum or urine of most patients with localized AL amyloidosis, even with sensitive assays. The course of localized AL amyloidosis is relatively benign, and treatment is generally confined to local surgical intervention, either alone or with radiotherapy, depending on the symptoms.

Systemic disease is more common than localized disease, and patients are often polysymptomatic at presentation (Table 10.2). Fatigue and weight loss are extremely common presenting symptoms but the diagnosis of amyloidosis is often delayed until dysfunction of a particular organ becomes apparent. The most common clinical findings at diagnosis include nephrotic syndrome, congestive cardiac failure and peripheral neuropathy. Although AL amyloid deposits

TABLE 10.2

Symptoms and clinical findings at presentation in patients with systemic AL amyloidosis

Symptoms	Clinical findings
• Fatigue	• Nephrotic syndrome (with or without renal insufficiency)
• Weight loss	
• Ankle swelling	• Congestive cardiac failure
• Lassitude	• Sensorimotor and/or autonomic neuropathy
• Breathlessness	
• Orthostatic hypotension	• Macroglossia (enlargement of the tongue)
	• Bruising
	• Hepatomegaly
	• Pleural infusions or occult pericardial effusions

generally affect multiple organs, dysfunction of one particular organ often predominates. Nearly 50% of patients have dominant renal amyloidosis at diagnosis, which usually presents as nephrotic syndrome due to a glomerular lesion. Substantial albuminuria in the context of myeloma, as opposed to isolated Bence Jones proteinuria, should alert the clinician to the possibility of AL amyloidosis.

A quarter of patients have dominant symptomatic cardiac amyloidosis at diagnosis, which confers a very poor prognosis. Reduced QRS voltages in the ECG may precede clinical congestive cardiac failure. Cardiomyopathy in amyloidosis is restrictive because of thickened cardiac walls. Clinical signs are mainly right-sided heart failure, arrhythmias or signs associated with a low cardiac output, including orthostatic hypotension.

Up to 15% of patients present with symptoms of an axonal length-dependent peripheral neuropathy, most commonly a peripheral symmetric sensory neuropathy, with paresthesias, numbness and possibly pain; motor neuropathy is rare. Carpal tunnel syndrome is common, and may predate other symptoms by over a year. Autonomic neuropathy typically leads to postural hypotension, weight loss and disturbed gastrointestinal motility, and is often associated with some degree of peripheral neuropathy. Other clinical manifestations of autonomic disorders may also be observed, including erectile dysfunction, altered bowel habit, early satiety and gustatory sweating.

Involvement of the gastrointestinal tract may be focal or diffuse, and symptoms reflect the site and extent of involvement. Enlargement of the tongue (macroglossia) occurs in about 10% of patients and is virtually pathognomonic of AL amyloidosis. Other features of gastrointestinal amyloid include early satiety, diarrhea, chronic nausea, malabsorption, weight loss, gut perforation and overt rectal bleeding. Approximately 25% of patients have hepatomegaly at diagnosis, and it can be challenging to differentiate hepatic amyloid infiltration from venous congestion.

Hemorrhage is a frequent manifestation of amyloidosis, and can be a serious chronic problem. An abnormal clotting screen is found in about 50% of patients with AL amyloidosis. The mechanism is often multifactorial and may include vascular fragility or depletion of

vitamin K-dependent clotting factors. Periorbital purpura is particularly characteristic. Less frequent manifestations of systemic AL amyloidosis include:
- skin and soft-tissue thickening
- lymphadenopathy
- painful seronegative arthropathy
- bone involvement
- vocal cord infiltration
- adrenal gland or thyroid infiltration resulting in hypoadrenalism or hypothyroidism
- pulmonary infiltration.

Diagnosis

A diagnostic pathway for AL amyloidosis is shown in Figure 10.3. The diagnosis is on histological grounds, based on Congo red staining of a biopsy sample from an affected organ: amyloid deposits produce a characteristic green birefringence when viewed under cross-polarized light. Alternatively, the diagnosis may be confirmed in suspected cases with 50–80% sensitivity by staining a subcutaneous abdominal fat aspirate, although a negative result does not exclude amyloid. When amyloid is identified, the fibril type (AL or AA) and the extent of organ involvement should be determined.

Immunohistochemical staining for Ig light chains in AL amyloidosis has only about 60% sensitivity, and the presence of a paraprotein in serum or urine does not, by itself, confirm a diagnosis of AL amyloidosis. Importantly, both hereditary and wild-type ATTR (senile systemic) are more common than previously thought and may coexist with MGUS, creating a risk of misdiagnosis and unnecessary exposure to chemotherapy. Immunohistochemical typing of amyloid is challenging; definitive results are obtained in fewer than 60% of patients with AL amyloidosis.

By contrast, immunohistochemistry can reliably confirm or exclude amyloidosis of AA and TTR types. Hereditary forms of systemic amyloidosis can be reliably diagnosed by identifying mutations in the genes for transthyretin, fibrinogen Aα chain, lysozyme, apolipoprotein A1 and A2, gelsolin, cystatin C and β_2-microglobulin.

AL amyloidosis

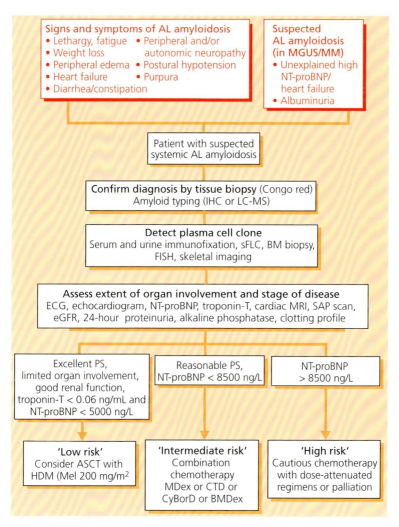

Figure 10.3 Diagnostic pathway for AL amyloidosis. ASCT, autologous stem-cell transplantation; BM, bone marrow; CyBorD, cyclophosphamide–bortezomib–dexamethasone; eGFR, estimated glomerular filtration rate; FISH, fluorescence in situ hybridization; FLC, free light chains; HDM, high-dose melphalan; IHC, immunohistochemistry; LC-MS, liquid chromatography mass spectrometry; MDex, melphalan–dexamethasone; MGUS, monoclonal gammopathy of undetermined significance; MM, multiple myeloma; MRI, magnetic resonance imaging; NT-proBNP, N-terminal pro-brain natriuretic peptide; PS, performance status, SAP, serum amyloid P.

Demonstration of bone marrow involvement by serum amyloid P component (SAP) scintigraphy is virtually diagnostic of AL; similarly, demonstration of a particular pattern of abnormal cardiac uptake on 3,3-diphosphono-1,2-propanodicarboxylic acid (DPD) scintigraphy is strongly suggestive of cardiac ATTR.

Immunohistochemical staining of amyloidotic tissue, with genetic sequencing where necessary, should be undertaken in all cases of amyloidosis. In selected cases where the diagnosis is uncertain, this should be followed by amyloid fibril sequencing or mass spectrometry.

Investigations for underlying plasma cell dyscrasia or B-cell non-Hodgkin lymphoma. Immunofixation of serum and urine, and measurement of serum free light chains (sFLC), should be performed in all patients with suspected AL amyloidosis. Patients usually have low levels of clonal protein (involved sFLC or paraprotein), although clonal protein is not detected in the serum or urine in a minority of cases. Bone marrow aspirate and trephine biopsy are useful for identifying MGUS, MM or B-cell non-Hodgkin lymphoma, including Waldenström's macroglobulinemia. Congo red staining of a bone marrow trephine biopsy can be useful to confirm the diagnosis of amyloidosis. Immunophenotyping of bone marrow by flow cytometry should be performed to confirm the clonality of plasma cells, or to identify a B-cell clone.

Assessment of organ function. The extent of amyloid involvement should be assessed before planning therapy. Radiolabeled SAP localizes rapidly and specifically to amyloid deposits in proportion to the quantity of amyloid present, and SAP scintigraphy is useful to identify systemic amyloid in organs other than the heart and nerves. Cardiac amyloid deposition is associated with characteristic ECG changes (low QRS voltages) which can provide useful diagnostic information. Echocardiographic features of amyloidosis include concentrically thickened ventricular walls, with normal or small ventricular cavities, preserved ejection fraction, thickened valves and dilated atria.

N-terminal pro-brain natriuretic peptide (NT-proBNP) and cardiac troponin T (TnT) concentrations may be elevated in patients with a history of cardiac conditions and chronic kidney disease. Both are elevated in the presence of significant cardiac amyloid deposition, and are prognostic. Subendocardial late gadolinium enhancement on cardiac MRI is highly characteristic of cardiac amyloid deposition, while ^{99}Tc-DPD scanning is sensitive for the detection of cardiac ATTR. Significant non-Bence Jones proteinuria, hepatomegaly with raised alkaline phosphatase, and axonal peripheral neuropathy often indicate renal, liver and nerve amyloid involvement, respectively.

Staging and prognosis

The survival of patients with AL amyloidosis has improved significantly in the last 5 years as a result of earlier diagnosis, better supportive care and improved chemotherapeutic strategies to suppress the neoplastic clone. Survival is clearly linked to the extent of amyloid involvement and the organ involved; cardiac involvement carries the worst prognosis. Levels of cardiac biomarkers (NT-proBNP and TnT) and sFLC measurements are used in current prognostic scoring systems, and are particularly useful for identifying patients with poor prognosis, for whom palliation may be the most appropriate treatment. The Mayo Clinic staging system[2] (Table 10.3) is widely used and is the gold standard for staging AL amyloidosis. Overall survival is estimated at more than 8 years for patients with stage I disease but only 12 and 6 months for patients with stage III and IV disease, respectively.

Clinical management

The management of patients with AL amyloidosis needs to be individualized according to the extent of organ involvement, age, performance status, underlying hematologic disorder and the patient's wishes. Often, the treatment program for AL amyloidosis is aligned with anti-myeloma or lymphoma therapies. Very few randomized trials have been performed in patients with newly diagnosed AL amyloidosis; most of the available data come from retrospective single-arm studies of treatment combinations in selected patients.

TABLE 10.3

The Mayo Clinic staging system for AL amyloidosis[2]

Disease stage	Score	1 point each for:
I	0	• Cardiac TnT ≥ 0.025 ng/mL
II	1	• NT-proBNP ≥ 1800 pg/mL
III	2	• FLC difference ≥ 180 mg/dL*
IV	3	

*Difference between involved and uninvolved free light chain (FLC).
NT-proBNP, N-terminal pro-brain natriuretic peptide; TnT, troponin.

Localized AL amyloidosis can be treated with surgical resection or, occasionally, radiotherapy, with good long-term outcomes.

Systemic AL amyloidosis. The aim of therapy is to achieve a durable clonal remission that leads to initial stabilization of amyloid deposition and gradual regression over several years.

High-dose melphalan and ASCT is the preferred first-line treatment for patients up to 65–70 years of age with an estimated glomerular filtration rate above 50 mL/min, low cardiac biomarkers and low plasma cell infiltration of the bone marrow at transplantation.[3] Patients with a performance status above 2, severe autonomic neuropathy, significant gastrointestinal bleeding due to amyloid, or recurrent pleural effusions due to pulmonary amyloid are not candidates for ASCT. Patients with plasma cell infiltration typical of MM may benefit from induction therapy prior to ASCT using agents that are not toxic to stem cells.

Non-transplant approaches. First-line treatment for patients who are not eligible for ASCT involves chemotherapy regimens similar to those used in MM, although dexamethasone is typically used at a reduced dose. Regimens based on proteasome inhibitors are preferred over immunomodulatory drugs in light of better clonal response rates and outcomes in Phase II studies; subcutaneous bortezomib with an alkylating agent and a steroid is preferred when a rapid response is desirable. Thalidomide should be used with caution in patients with cardiac stage III disease or grade 3–4 neuropathy. Doses of all therapies may require modification given the higher treatment-related toxicity in patients with AL amyloidosis.

Relapsed disease. There are no standard treatments in this situation; re-treatment with initial therapies can be considered if a long sustained response was obtained previously. On the basis of single-arm Phase II studies, lenalidomide at reduced doses and pomalidomide can be considered for relapsed disease.

Monitoring of response. FLC, M protein or both should be measured after each cycle of chemotherapy and every 2–3 months following therapy discontinuation; an early switch to an alternative regimen may be beneficial in some patients who do not respond to treatment. The difference between the involved and uninvolved light chain (dFLC) should be used to monitor hematologic response, provided the dFLC is more than 50 mg/L at diagnosis. M protein can be used if it is greater than 5 g/L. Echocardiography, NT-proBNP measurement and cardiac MRI can be used to monitor cardiac response. Routine measurements of renal function, including creatinine clearance and 24-hour urine protein excretion, urine protein-creatinine ratio or both, give a good assessment of renal response.[4] Organ and hematologic response criteria are summarized in Table 10.4.

Supportive care

Congestive cardiac failure should be managed symptomatically using diuretics; selected patients with cardiac amyloidosis may benefit from appropriate cardiac device therapy to improve cardiac function. Young patients with predominant cardiac amyloidosis and good clonal response to induction therapy should be considered for cardiac transplantation. In some patients, orthostatic hypotension may respond to the use of support stockings, together with modest doses of fludrocortisone; midodrine may be more effective in patients with amyloidosis but can cause supine hypertension. Renal transplantation may be considered for selected patients with renal amyloidosis and renal failure on hemodialysis. Nutritional supplementation may be required for patients with gastrointestinal amyloidosis.

TABLE 10.4

Criteria for organ and hematologic response

Organ	Response	Progression
Heart	NT-proBNP response (> 30% and > 35 pmol/L decrease in patients with baseline NT-proBNP ≥ 77 pmol/L) or NYHA class response (≥ 2 class decrease in patients with baseline NYHA class 3 or 4)	NT-proBNP progression (> 30% and > 35 pmol/L increase)* or Cardiac TnT progression (≥ 33% increase), or Ejection fraction progression (≥ 10% decrease)
Kidney	50% decrease (≥ 0.5 g/day) in 24-hour urine protein (urine protein must be > 0.5 g/day pretreatment) Creatinine and creatinine clearance must not worsen by 25% over baseline	50% increase (≥ 1 g/day) in 24-hour urine protein to > 1 g/day or 25% worsening of serum creatinine or creatinine clearance
Liver	50% decrease in abnormal alkaline phosphatase value Decrease in liver size on radiography of ≥ 2 cm	50% increase of alkaline phosphatase above the lowest value
Peripheral nervous system	Improvement in electromyogram nerve conduction velocity (rare)	Progressive neuropathy by electromyography or nerve conduction velocity
Hematologic	PR: 50% reduction in dFLC VGPR: reduction in dFLC to < 40 mg/L CR: normal FLC levels with normal κ/λ ratio and negative serum and urine immunofixation for M protein	

*Patients with progressively worsening renal function cannot be scored for NT-ProBNP progression.
CR, complete response; dFLC, difference between the involved and uninvolved FLC; FLC, free light chain; NHYA, New York Heart Association; NT-proBNP, N-terminal pro-brain natriuretic peptide; PR, partial response; TnT, troponin; VGPR, very good partial response.

Key points – AL amyloidosis

- AL amyloidosis is a rare multisystem hematologic disorder caused by an underlying plasma cell dyscrasia.
- Local amyloidosis can be managed with surgery or radiotherapy, with good long-term outcomes.
- Systemic AL amyloidosis is staged according to the degree of cardiac involvement and serum free light chains.
- Autologous stem cell transplantation is the treatment of choice for selected patients with AL amyloidosis.
- Proteasome inhibitor-based therapy is preferred in newly diagnosed patients; immunomodulator-based therapy is often used after relapse.

References

1. Gertz M. Immunoglobulin light chain amyloidosis: 2013 update on diagnosis, prognosis, and treatment. *Am J Hematol* 2013;88:416–25.

2. Kumar S, Dispenzieri A, Lacy MQ et al. Revised prognostic staging system for light chain amyloidosis incorporating cardiac biomarkers and serum free light chain measurements. *J Clin Oncol* 2012;30:989–95.

3. Cordes S, Dispenzieri A, Lacy MQ et al. Ten-year survival after autologous stem cell transplantation for immunoglobulin light chain amyloidosis. *Cancer* 2012;118:6105–109.

4. Palladini G, Dispenzieri A, Gertz MA et al. New criteria for response to treatment in immunoglobulin light chain amyloidosis based on free light chain measurement and cardiac biomarkers: impact on survival outcomes. *J Clin Oncol* 2012;30:4541–9.

11 Rare plasma cell dyscrasias

In addition to multiple myeloma (MM), a number of rare plasma cell dyscrasias may be encountered in clinical practice:
- plasmacytoma
- Waldenström's macroglobulinemia (WM)
- POEMS (polyneuropathy, organomegaly, endocrinopathy, monoclonal gammopathy and skin changes) syndrome.

Plasmacytoma

Plasmacytoma is a rare localized tumor that accounts for fewer than 10% of all plasma cell neoplasms. Plasmacytomas most commonly occur with MM, as solitary or multiple tumors in medullary or extramedullary locations (Table 11.1; Figure 11.1); plasmacytomas of bone or soft tissues are less common in the absence of MM. Plasmacytomas presenting with intramedullary myeloma are managed in the same way as MM, and are not discussed further.

Clinical presentation. Patients with plasmacytoma present with bone pain or fractures. The plasmacytoma is often in the spine or pelvis, although long bones or ribs may occasionally be affected; in rare cases, a biopsy of soft tissue or bone lumps can lead to an incidental diagnosis of plasmacytoma. Patients may also present to the emergency department with spinal cord compression secondary to a solitary spinal plasmacytoma. Blood count and biochemical profiles

TABLE 11.1
Classification of plasmacytomas

- Solitary plasmacytoma
- Solitary plasmacytoma with bone marrow involvement
- Multifocal plasmacytoma without bone marrow involvement

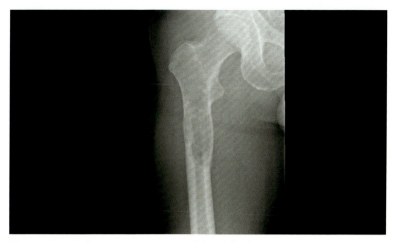

Figure 11.1 Solitary plasmacytoma of the right femur.

are often normal, and clonal protein levels in serum and/or urine may be low. Pain relief and stabilization of the affected bone are required before further investigation.

Extramedullary plasmacytomas are less common than solitary bone plasmacytomas, and present as infiltration of the soft tissue by clonal plasma cells. More than 80% of extramedullary plasmacytomas are found in the head and neck region, particularly the upper respiratory tract; the gastrointestinal tract is the next most frequent site. Tumors are usually localized, and progression to MM is rare. In contrast to solitary bone plasmacytomas, monoclonal protein is detected in serum or urine in fewer than 25% of patients with extramedullary plasmacytomas.

Multiple plasmacytomas occur in up to 5% of patients and may involve soft tissue or bone, but with no evidence of bone marrow involvement. Such cases usually have a indolent course and rarely progress to MM.

Diagnosis and follow-up. The initial diagnostic work-up should include a full blood count with blood film examination to exclude anemia, and biochemical screening, including renal, liver and bone profiles, to exclude renal dysfunction and hypercalcemia. Serum immunoglobulin (Ig) levels, serum protein electrophoresis and immunofixation and a serum free light chain (sFLC) assay usually highlight low-level clonal protein; higher sFLC is a risk factor for early progression to MM in patients with solitary plasmacytoma. Urine protein electrophoresis and immunofixation may also be positive in a small proportion of patients.

A full skeletal survey, whole body FDG-PET-CT and MRI of the spine and pelvis are warranted if the patient has back or pelvic pain. MRI is useful in characterizing vertebral and spinal lesions, and aids the planning of radiotherapy, with or without vertebral augmentation. Whole-body PET-CT helps to identify multiple plasmacytomas in bony or extramedullary locations (Figure 11.2); the risk of progression to MM is higher in patients with multiple plasmacytomas with bone marrow involvement. Bone marrow aspirate and trephine biopsy with plasma cell phenotyping should be performed in all patients in order to identify those with bone marrow involvement (up to 70% of patients), as this is associated with a higher risk of progression to MM.[1] The possibility of plasmacytoma associated with intramedullary myeloma should be excluded before treatment is initiated.

During follow-up, serum protein electrophoresis and immunofixation plus sFLC measurement can detect early recurrence or progression in patients with plasmacytoma; whole-body PET-CT

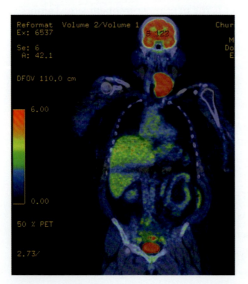

Figure 11.2

Extramedullary plasmacytoma: PET scan of a solitary plasmacytoma of the thyroid.

should be considered if patients report symptoms. Routine follow-up imaging or bone marrow examination is not advisable in asymptomatic patients.

Management

Solitary bone plasmacytoma. Definitive therapy should be planned because cure can be achieved in a small proportion of patients. Radical radiotherapy is the treatment of choice, based on retrospective studies that have shown excellent local disease control with radiotherapy alone. Radiotherapy should encompass the tumor volume seen on MRI, plus a margin of at least 2 cm; the normal dose is 40 Gy given over 20 fractions although a higher dose of 50 Gy in 25 fractions can be considered for tumors larger than 5 cm. A single trial found adjuvant chemotherapy to be effective in preventing relapse; further trials are required to determine whether patients at higher risk of relapse or progression can be identified. Relapse often occurs outside the initial radiation field but local recurrence has also been reported. Progression to myeloma may occur in patients with bone marrow involvement at diagnosis following radiotherapy to the index lesion alone. Some patients may require surgical fixation of a solitary bone plasmacytoma.

Extramedullary plasmacytoma should be treated with radical radiotherapy, as cure rates of up to 90% have been reported in single-center retrospective studies. As with solitary bone plasmacytoma, the radiotherapy field should include the primary tumor plus a 2 cm margin, and any involved cervical nodes. The radiotherapy dosage is the same as for solitary bone plasmacytoma. For selected patients with large plasmacytomas where the radiotherapy field is unlikely to safely cover the tumor site, chemotherapy or surgery can be considered, either before or after radiotherapy. Surgical resection of soft tissue followed by adjuvant radiotherapy may be recommended in a few patients.

Multifocal plasmacytoma. The choice of therapy for these patients will be influenced by age, number of lesions, and the disease-free interval in those with recurrent disease. Patients with more extensive disease or early relapse after radiotherapy may benefit from systemic therapy alone or with autologous stem cell transplantation (ASCT), as in the treatment of MM. In the absence of systemic disease, recurrent solitary plasmacytoma at sites remote from the original site of radiotherapy can be treated with additional radiotherapy, with good long-term results.

Waldenström's macroglobulinemia

WM is a low-grade lymphoproliferative disorder characterized by infiltration of lymphoplasmacytoid in the bone marrow and elevated IgM production. It is a rare disorder, with an annual incidence of 0.55 per 100 000 in the UK, and predominantly affects men. Between 1000 and 1500 cases of WM are diagnosed annually in the USA (3 per million per year). The median age at presentation is over 70 years, and median survival is about 5 years.

WM is preceded by a benign phase of monoclonal gammopathy of undetermined significance (MGUS) dominated by IgM production. Population-based studies have shown an increased risk of WM and IgM MGUS in first-degree relatives of patients with WM. Patients and their first-degree relatives appear to have a shared susceptibility for autoimmune diseases and WM.

Clinical features. The majority of patients with WM are asymptomatic and require infrequent monitoring. Clinical features in symptomatic patients are primarily related to disease burden and include:
- fatigue
- breathlessness
- peripheral neuropathy
- organomegaly
- cytopenias
- frequent infections
- weight loss.

In addition, associated plasma hyperviscosity syndrome, amyloidosis, cold hemagglutinin disease (CHAD) and acquired von Willebrand disease can lead to a distinct set of symptoms in up to 25% of patients, including headaches, breathlessness, cardiac failure, hemolysis and bleeding. Bing–Neel syndrome is a rare central nervous comorbidity associated with cognitive decline, cranial nerve involvement, seizures and headaches.

Pathophysiology. WM is caused by accumulation in the marrow and lymphatic regions of post-germinal center cells that have undergone somatic hypermutation under the influence of antigen selection, without isotype switching (see Chapter 3). Gene expression profiling (GEP) suggests that these cells are more closely related to malignant mature B cells than to plasma cells. Deletion of chromosome 6q is the most frequent cytogenetic abnormality in WM, occurring in 50% of cases; however, the influence of this genetic change on clinical outcomes is unclear. Deletion of the *p53* gene is seen in a small number of patients and is associated with poor outcomes. Whole genome sequencing has demonstrated a single point mutation, L265P, in the myeloid differentiation primary response gene (*MYD88*) in 90% of patients with WM. This mutation appears to be a useful marker to distinguish between WM and marginal zone non-Hodgkin lymphoma, and has also been reported in patients with IgM MGUS.

Diagnosis. Patients presenting with IgM paraprotein, with or without symptoms, should be investigated to identify IgM MGUS or asymptomatic or symptomatic WM. Investigations for the diagnosis of WM are summarized in Table 11.2. Clinical features such as plasma hyperviscosity, recurrent headaches, retinal changes, bleeding and breathlessness should be evaluated, and comorbidities assessed, in order to determine suitability for any planned therapy and to identify features of high-grade transformation.

The presence of cytopenias could reflect a heavy marrow burden or hypersplenism, while the presence of high IgM levels or excessive light chain production could indicate renal impairment. Amyloidosis should be suspected in patients with neuropathy, raised alkaline phosphatase or significant proteinuria. Hepatitis testing is useful in patients with associated cryoglobulins and for those in whom B-cell-depleting therapies are planned. Lymphadenopathy and splenomegaly are present in up to 15% of patients and can be assessed by CT scanning. Trephine biopsy provides the best means of assessing marrow burden.

TABLE 11.2

Investigations for the diagnosis of Waldenström's macroglobulinemia

- Full blood count
- Plasma viscosity
- Serum protein electrophoresis and immunofixation
- Serum free light chain assay
- Renal profile
- Liver function tests
- Lactate dehydrogenase
- β_2-microglobulin
- Direct antiglobulin test
- Urine protein/creatinine ratio
- Hepatitis B and C status
- Anti-myelin-associated glycoprotein titer
- Nerve conduction studies
- Cold agglutinins
- Cryoglobulins
- Bone marrow aspirate and trephine biopsy with flow cytometry and metaphase karyotyping
- CT of the chest/abdomen/pelvis

Flow cytometry is helpful to identify the B-cell clone and to discriminate WM from marginal zone lymphoma.

Clinical outcomes for patients with WM vary significantly so it is important to identify the level of risk. The international prognostic scoring system for WM stratifies risk as low, intermediate or high according to age, hemoglobin concentration, platelet count, and β_2-microglobulin and paraprotein concentrations (Table 11.3).

Management of patients with newly diagnosed and relapsed WM. Many patients with WM are asymptomatic at diagnosis, and infrequent monitoring (every 4 months) for symptoms and changes

TABLE 11.3

The international prognostic scoring system for Waldenström's macroglobulinemia[3]

Each factor scores 1 point

- Age > 65 years
- Hemoglobin < 11.5 g/dL
- Platelet count < 100 × 10^9/L
- β_2-microglobulin > 3 mg/L
- Monoclonal IgM > 7.0 g/dL

Risk level	Score (points)	5-year survival
Low	0 or 1 (except age)	87%
Intermediate	2 or age	68%
High	≥ 3	36%

in blood variables is recommended. The 5-year risk of progression from asymptomatic to symptomatic WM is 59%. Indications for therapy are:

- constitutional symptoms such as weight loss, night sweats, fevers
- symptomatic lymphadenopathy or splenomegaly
- plasma hyperviscosity
- marrow suppression due to infiltration
- peripheral neuropathy and associated CHAD or amyloidosis.

Plasma hyperviscosity (> 4 centipoise) at diagnosis reflects the fact that 80% of IgM is intravascular. Therapeutic plasma exchange is recommended to reduce high plasma viscosity, lower IgM concentrations and reverse the clinical effects of hyperviscosity. A single-volume plasma exchange reduces IgM levels by approximately 40% and plasma viscosity by 60%.

Patients with WM are often elderly and have multiple comorbidities. A comprehensive assessment of frailty, organ function and performance status is therefore required before treatment is decided. Given that WM is an incurable low-grade lymphoproliferative disorder, a palliative approach may be reasonable in frail patients with poor performance status.

Evidence-based management of WM is challenging, given a lack of Phase III trial data. The response to therapy is assessed primarily from the decrease in IgM monoclonal protein achieved (minimal response > 25% decrease; partial response > 50% decrease; very good partial response > 90% decrease); complete response requires confirmation of no residual plasma or lymphoplasmacytoid cells in the bone marrow. CT scans showing partial or complete resolution of lymphadenopathy and splenomegaly are required for responses graded as partial remission and above.

In Phase III trials in patients with newly diagnosed and relapsed WM, fludarabine monotherapy has been found to be more effective than comparators (chlorambucil or cyclophosphamide–vincristine–prednisolone [COP]), in terms of response rates and progression-free survival. Although not tested in Phase III trials, rituximab, as monotherapy or in combination with DNA-damaging chemotherapeutic agents (fludarabine, cyclophosphamide), has improved response rates. Single-arm Phase II trials of bortezomib with rituximab showed rapid responses and objective response rates of up to 80%, but high neuropathy rates; randomized trials are investigating weekly subcutaneous bortezomib therapy. It is recommended that patients with newly diagnosed symptomatic WM receive a rituximab-containing regimen such as:[2]

- rituximab, cyclophosphamide and dexamethasone (RCD)
- bendamustine and rituximab (BR)
- fludarabine and rituximab (FR)
- fludarabine, cyclophosphamide and rituximab (FCR).

The choice of regimen should take into consideration performance status, clinical features such as renal function, comorbidities and potential eligibility for stem cell transplantation (Figure 11.3).[3] Given the risk of IgM flare (a marked but transient increase in IgM production following initiation of treatment), the introduction of rituximab should be deferred in patients with hyperviscosity or high IgM protein levels (> 4 g/dL). Ibrutinib (a Bruton tyrosine kinase inhibitor) is licensed for use in patients with newly diagnosed WM where chemoimmunotherapy is contraindicated, and is being explored in trials.

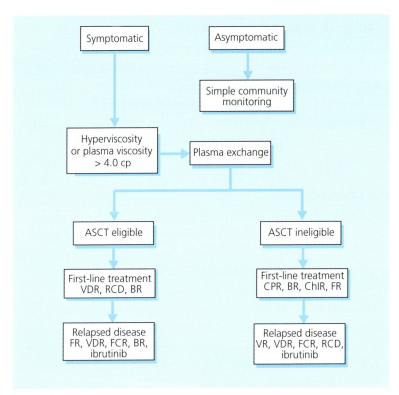

Figure 11.3 Treatment pathway for Waldenström's macroglobulinemia. ASCT, autologous stem cell transplantation; BR, bendamustine–rituximab; ChlR, chlorambucil–rituximab; cp, centipoise; CPR, cyclophosphamide–prednisone–rituximab; FCR, fludarabine–cyclophosphamide–rituximab; FR, fludarabine–rituximab; RCD, rituximab–cyclophosphamide–dexamethasone; VR, bortezomib–rituximab; VDR, bortezomib–dexamethasone–rituximab.

Ibrutinib has also recently been approved as monotherapy for patients with relapsed symptomatic WM in light of a significantly high objective response rate of 87% in a single-arm open-label study. Re-treatment with the same regimen can be considered if a durable response (more than 2 years) is achieved with initial therapy. Re-induction with either bendamustine or bortezomib in combination with rituximab can also be considered. Consolidation with ASCT to enhance the durability of response should be considered in suitable patients.

Allogeneic stem cell transplantation is an option in young, fit, chemotherapy-sensitive patients with a fully matched donor. Patients with high-grade transformation (biopsy-proven diffuse large B cell lymphoma [DLBCL]) should receive intensive chemotherapy as recommended in primary DLBCL treatment protocols. Supportive care with prophylactic anti-infective agents and vaccination against Pneumococcus spp, *Haemophilus influenzae* and viral influenza is recommended.

POEMS syndrome

POEMS syndrome describes a cluster of polyradiculoneuropathy, organomegaly, endocrinopathy, skin changes and monoclonal protein secondary to an underlying plasma cell clone. The diagnosis of this syndrome is often delayed because the predominant neuropathy may be erroneously ascribed to a neurological disorder, most commonly chronic inflammatory demyelinating polyneuropathy. The pathogenesis of the syndrome is poorly understood, and prognosis and management are based on clinical phenotype rather than disease-specific markers. POEMS syndrome often overlaps with Castleman disease and osteosclerotic myeloma.

Clinical features. Criteria for the diagnosis of POEMS syndrome are summarized in Table 11.4. Neuropathic symptoms are the dominant feature; sclerotic bone lesions are usually asymptomatic. Predominant symptoms may also be those of associated endocrinopathy, particularly adrenal and gonadal dysfunction. Symptomatic organomegaly can often limit mobility and exercise tolerance. Skin lesions (hypertrichosis and hemangiomas) and ocular symptoms, such as blurred vision due to papilledema, may also be present. In addition, up to 20% of patients have venous or arterial thrombotic events.

Investigations. The diagnosis of POEMS syndrome is based on a combination of clinicopathological features. Monoclonal protein is restricted to lambda (λ) light chains in the majority of patients. The full blood count may be normal, although polycythemia or thrombocytosis may be present and are linked to underlying disease

TABLE 11.4

Diagnostic criteria for POEMS syndrome

Diagnosis of POEMS syndrome is confirmed when both of the mandatory major criteria, one of the three other major criteria, and one of the six minor criteria are present.

Mandatory major criteria	• Polyneuropathy (typically demyelinating) • Monoclonal plasma cell-proliferative disorder (almost always λ)
Other major criteria (one required)	• Castleman disease • Sclerotic bone lesions • Elevated VEGF
Minor criteria (one required)	• Organomegaly (splenomegaly, hepatomegaly or lymphadenopathy) • Extravascular volume overload (edema, pleural effusion or ascites) • Endocrinopathy (adrenal, thyroid [except hypothyroidism]), pituitary, gonadal, parathyroid and pancreatic [except diabetes]) • Skin changes (hyperpigmentation, hypertrichosis, glomeruloid hemangiomata, plethora, acrocyanosis, flushing and white nails) • Papilledema • Thrombocytosis/polycythemia
Other symptoms and signs	• Clubbing • Weight loss • Hyperhidrosis • Pulmonary manifestations • Hypertension/restrictive lung disease • Thrombotic diatheses • Diarrhea • Low vitamin B_{12} values

VEGF, vascular endothelial growth factor.

activity. Nerve conduction studies are required to assess the extent and type of neuropathy. An endocrinopathy screen, echocardiogram and lung function tests are also required. Serum concentrations of vascular endothelial growth factor (VEGF) can be a good marker of disease activity and should be measured at baseline and every 3 months thereafter. Serum and urine protein electrophoresis, immunofixation and sFLC can be useful to detect low levels of monoclonal protein. Bone marrow biopsy is crucial to identify the plasma cell clone, and characteristic lymphoid nodules can be observed; megakaryocyte hyperplasia and clustering have also been reported. Skeletal radiography and whole-body PET-CT are useful to determine the extent and location of sclerotic lesions and suitability for radiotherapy.

It is important to distinguish POEMS syndrome from MGUS, solitary plasmacytoma and smoldering myeloma with neuropathy, because the management, supportive care and disease course differ.

Management. Given the rarity of the condition, randomized trials have not been performed in POEMS syndrome. The exact incidence is unknown, with large centers managing fewer than 100 patients. Hence, treatment options are primarily guided by retrospective case series.[4] The choice of treatment depends on the extent of disease, as assessed by the presence of clonal plasma cells on bone marrow biopsy and the number of bone lesions at diagnosis.
- Patients with no clonal cells in the marrow biopsy and a single focal bone lesion can be managed with localized radiotherapy.
- For patients with multifocal bone lesions and disseminated marrow involvement, systemic therapy based on experience in other plasma cell dyscrasias is used.
- For patients who are eligible for transplantation, high-dose melphalan conditioning is followed by stem cell rescue. Durable responses, with improvement in neuropathy, have been observed several months after transplant. However, an engraftment syndrome can occur, consisting of rash, fever, respiratory deterioration and weight gain, necessitating steroid treatment. An increased transfusion requirement has also been reported in patients with splenomegaly.

- In patients who are not transplant candidates, melphalan or cyclophosphamide can be used in combination with steroids, with good hematologic and organ function responses. Lenalidomide in combination with dexamethasone appears to be effective in the treatment of both newly diagnosed and relapsed POEMS syndrome. This regimen is well tolerated, except for a rash and a high risk of thrombosis, which must be managed with adequate thromboprophylaxis. Thalidomide- and bortezomib-based therapies are associated with a risk of neurotoxicity and are therefore not advised in patients with POEMS syndrome. A few reports have demonstrated clinical responses with bevacizumab (anti-VEGF therapy).

Reduction in clonal protein can be observed in response to treatment and can be used to monitor relapse. In addition, organ responses, such as reductions in neuropathy and third space collection (ascites, pleural effusion, pedal edema), have occasionally been observed in patients with residual clonal protein: such responses are primarily assessed on clinical grounds, although VEGF levels can be a useful marker of disease activity in these patients.

Key points – rare plasma cell dyscrasias

- Solitary medullary or extramedullary plasmacytoma is a curable disorder.
- Multifocal plasmacytoma is best managed using the multiple myeloma treatment pathway.
- Waldenström's macroglobulinemia (WM) is an incurable low-grade B-cell lymphoproliferative neoplasm presenting at about 70 years of age and may be asymptomatic.
- Rituximab-based combination therapy is suitable for both newly diagnosed and relapsed WM in patients with good performance.
- POEMS syndrome is a rare multisystem plasma cell dyscrasia due solely to lambda light chains, and is dominated by peripheral neuropathy.

Patients require considerable supportive care because of reduced mobility secondary to neuropathy and severe generalized edema (anasarca). Patients benefit from physiotherapy, which should be organized in parallel with systemic therapy. Oxygen supplementation has been shown to improve quality of life in patients with poor pulmonary reserve.

References

1. Hill QA, Rawstron AC, deTute RM, Owen RG. Outcome prediction in plasmacytoma of bone: a risk model utilizing bone marrow flow cytometry and light-chain analysis. *Blood* 2014;124:1296–9.

2. Dimopoulos M, Kastritis E, Owen RG et al. Treatment recommendations for patients with Waldenström macroglobulinaemia (WM) and related disorders: IWWM-7 consensus. *Blood* 2014;124:1404–11.

3. Morel P, Duhamel A, Gobbi P et al. International prognostic scoring system for Waldenstrom macroglobulinaemia. *Blood* 2009;113:4163–70.

4. Dispenzieri A. How I treat POEMS syndrome. *Blood* 2012;119:5650–8.

12 Supportive care

Survival in multiple myeloma (MM) has almost tripled over the past 10 years, and it is now projected that a third of patients will survive more than 10 years after diagnosis. Supportive care is essential to enhance long-term outcomes and improve quality of life; the key domains relate to disease activity, complications from anti-myeloma therapy and subsequent disease progression (Table 12.1).[1] Patients should be offered the support of an advanced nurse practitioner, and referral to other specialists should be considered when patients require ongoing support and symptoms are not adequately addressed.

It should be remembered that MM remains incurable, and patients eventually reach the end of life with relapsed or refractory disease, which requires careful management to ensure dignity in the last days and weeks.

Anemia

Up to three-quarters of patients with MM present with anemia, and others develop it during the course of the illness. Although rarely severe, anemia increases the fatigue that patients often experience while on chemotherapy, and worsens quality of life.

TABLE 12.1

Complications of multiple myeloma

- Bone disease
- Renal impairment
- Infection
- Anemia
- Pain
- Neuropathy
- Coagulation disorders

The cause of anemia is multifactorial. It may be related to comorbidities in elderly patients, heavy marrow infiltration, renal impairment, or increased hepcidin expression, reducing the availability of iron to erythrocytes. Furthermore, anemia can be worsened by chemotherapy, requiring close monitoring. Anemia is often normocytic but iron deficiency and bleeding should be excluded as possible causes.

Asymptomatic mild or moderate anemia secondary to MM can be managed simply with observation, and some patients will become less anemic as the myeloma is controlled with therapy. Moderate symptomatic anemia can be managed with blood transfusion or erythropoietin with supplemental iron therapy; blood transfusion can also be helpful in the short-term correction of moderate-to-severe anemia in symptomatic patients. Erythropoietin is recommended for anemia associated with renal impairment. Typical regimens include:

- darbepoetin, 6.25 µg/kg every 3 weeks
- epoetin alfa, 40 000 IU once weekly
- epoetin beta, 30 000 IU once weekly.

Doubling of the dose after 4 weeks can be considered in patients with a hemoglobin increase of less than 1.0 g/dL, but erythropoietin treatment should be stopped after 6–8 weeks if a hemoglobin response is not observed. Care is required to ensure that the hemoglobin concentration does not rise above 12.0 g/dL, which increases the risk of thrombosis. Use of erythropoietin appears to be safe in patients with MM who are receiving chemotherapy (at any stage of treatment).

Bone pain

Bone disease is often the presenting feature in patients with MM; the pathophysiology and management are described in Chapter 9. Bone pain is associated with significant morbidity, and limits everyday activities. The location and severity of pain should be assessed at diagnosis and follow-up visits: a visual analog scale (VAS) can be used to rate pain levels during follow-up.

Skeletal radiography and MRI of the whole spine and pelvis should be performed to assess structural damage to bone. It is important to distinguish between neuropathic pain arising from radiculopathy and myeloma-related bone pain.

Anti-myeloma therapy is the single most important tool to control associated bone pain, although radiotherapy, orthopedic procedures and vertebroplasty or kyphoplasty may be appropriate to alleviate pain in some patients. Concomitant treatment with bisphosphonates and anti-myeloma therapy in responding patients often significantly decreases pain scores within the first 2 months. Often, however, cancer pain requires a multimodal approach involving opioids, calcium-channel blockers, sodium-channel blockers and norepinephrine-reuptake inhibitors; this may require liaison with a palliative care team or pain specialist. Regular use of non-steroidal anti-inflammatory drugs (NSAIDs) should be avoided because of the potential for renal toxicity.

Paracetamol (acetaminophen), 1 g four times daily, can be a useful non-opiate analgesic to control cancer-related pain. For patients with chronic mild-to-moderate pain (< 5 on a 10-point VAS) who do not respond to regular paracetamol, oral tramadol can be used on an as-required basis, increasing to regular treatment at a maximum dose of 100 mg/day four times daily. If pain remains uncontrolled, or the patient does not tolerate tramadol, codeine phosphate, 30 mg four times daily, can be used.

Oxycodone or morphine preparations are recommended for patients with chronic moderate-to-severe bone pain (> 5/10). Fast-acting preparations can be used to achieve initial control of pain, after which a sustained-release preparation can be considered, depending on the severity of pain, the response to treatment, dosage required and adverse effects. Fentanyl or buprenorphine patches can be considered if pain remains uncontrolled; these are often preferred by patients and have fewer side effects than other opiate preparations.

Subcutaneous oxycodone or morphine can be used to achieve rapid pain control in an acute situation; patients can be switched to long-term therapies as described above. Parenteral administration may be appropriate in special circumstances, such as for patients with reduced consciousness.

While opiate treatment provides effective pain control, patients should be monitored for side effects such as pruritus, constipation, emesis and excessive sedation.

More information on chronic pain management can be found in *Fast Facts: Chronic and Cancer Pain*.[4]

Infection

Up to 10% of patients with MM die prematurely, and a large proportion of these deaths are due to infections. Patients may be at high risk of infections because of defective humoral and cell-mediated immunity and bone disease, which leads to poor respiratory reserve and mobility. Although patients with myeloma do not have neutropenia, exposure to high doses of steroids – which are the mainstay of therapy together with immunomodulators and proteasome inhibitors – augments the risk. The use of prophylactic antibacterial agents has been limited by antibiotic resistance and *Clostridium difficile* infections, and evidence supporting prophylactic use of immunoglobulin infusions in myeloma patients remains contradictory. Polyvalent pneumococcal and *H. influenzae* vaccinations are recommended, although efficacy may vary according to the disease course. Patients should be offered information about the risk of infection and advised who to contact if they experience symptoms consistent with an active infection.

High-dose therapy and autologous stem cell transplantation (ASCT) may be complicated by bacterial sepsis secondary to chemotherapy-induced mucositis and bacterial translocation. However, the risk of fungal infections is significantly lower in patients with myeloma than in patients with myeloid malignancies undergoing intensive chemotherapy. Known risk factors for fungal infection include:
- high-dose steroid treatment
- graft versus host disease
- prolonged neutropenia.

Viral infection and reactivation is common in patients with MM, particularly in those undergoing ASCT. Herpes virus infections are common in the induction and post-transplantation phases of treatment but the risk can be significantly reduced by prophylaxis with aciclovir (acyclovir) and valaciclovir (valacyclovir). Treatment with proteasome inhibitors is also associated with an increased risk of herpes virus infection.

Neuropathy

Peripheral neuropathy is part of the initial presentation in a minority of patients with MM, and involvement of the central nervous system is rare. Neuropathy can be related to coexisting medical conditions such as hypothyroidism, diabetes, renal impairment, carpal tunnel syndrome or vitamin B_{12} deficiency. Typical neuropathy symptoms in patients with MM are summarized in Table 12.2. Treatment may make symptoms worse, or put patients at risk of emergent neuropathy. Baseline clinical assessment of neuropathy and neurophysiological testing are recommended.

Compressive neuropathies and radiculopathies. Spinal cord compression is a rare emergency presentation of MM that requires urgent radiotherapy, surgery or both to improve neurological outcomes. Vertebral involvement with fractures often leads to spinal cord compression, radiculopathy, or both; steroid treatment and liaison with a spinal surgical team is essential in such cases. Concomitant chemotherapy and radiotherapy can improve outcomes when started promptly, although patients may experience residual pain or weakness in the legs, requiring rehabilitation.

Peripheral neuropathy. Up to 20% of patients have documented peripheral neuropathy at diagnosis, which is usually subclinical. POEMS (polyneuropathy, organomegaly, endocrinopathy, monoclonal gammopathy and skin changes) syndrome and amyloid light-chain (AL) amyloidosis are established causes of peripheral neuropathy in patients with plasma cell dyscrasias. In addition, there is an association between monoclonal gammopathy of undetermined significance (MGUS), particularly IgM MGUS, and peripheral neuropathy. This often presents with insidious onset of progressive, symmetric, distal sensory or motor neuropathy with paresthesias and numbness; neurophysiological tests reveal a demyelinating neuropathy. Management of such neuropathy

TABLE 12.2
Neuropathy symptoms in patients with multiple myeloma

Sensory
- Sensation of wearing an invisible glove or sock
- Wooden quality
- Numbness, pins and needles
- Feeling of walking on pebbles
- Feelings of tightness and swelling
- Burning sensations, or freezing pain
- Sharp, jabbing or electric shock-like pain
- Extreme sensitivity to touch
- Loss of balance and coordination
- Cramps in the feet and legs

Motor
- Tripping on the toes
- Loss of grip strength

Autonomic
- Orthostatic dizziness
- Constipation
- Diarrhea
- Urinary incontinence
- Sexual dysfunction
- Dry eyes
- Dry mouth

often requires close liaison with neurologists, and some patients require treatment to suppress the plasma cell clone or to reduce M protein or autoantibody levels.

Treatment-induced neuropathy. Vinca alkaloids are well known to cause neuropathic symptoms in patients with hematologic malignancies and are no longer used in patients with MM.

Both thalidomide and bortezomib cause varying degrees of emergent neuropathy in patients with MM, and symptoms of peripheral and autonomic neuropathy (see Table 12.2) should be sought during treatment. Newer proteasome inhibitors ixazomib and carfilzomib are both associated with a significantly lower risk of neuropathy.

Thalidomide. Peripheral neuropathy may arise after prolonged administration of thalidomide (usually more than 6 months): this is mostly mild to moderate in severity and appears to be cumulative. Initial symptoms include sensory changes, such as paresthesia and hyperesthesia, followed by motor symptoms (weakness) and autonomic dysfunction. Later effects include loss of vibration and joint position sense, which leads to ataxia and progressive gait disturbance, with a high risk of falls. Nerve conduction studies do not predict significant peripheral neuropathy or correlate with clinical findings. Close monitoring and reduction or temporary discontinuation of thalidomide usually leads to a clinical improvement in symptoms, whereas continuation of intensive treatment in patients with peripheral neuropathy can cause permanent neurological damage.

Bortezomib-induced peripheral neuropathy is characterized by neuropathic pain and distal sensory neuropathy with suppression of reflexes. Motor neuropathy may follow, and occasionally results in distal weakness in the legs. Patients may report significant autonomic neuropathy, which manifests as dizziness, hypotension, diarrhea or constipation, and extreme fatigue. Neuropathy may develop early in the course of treatment, or may be delayed. Neurophysiological testing reveals a distal sensorimotor axonal loss, with secondary demyelination.

Symptoms usually improve or resolve within 3 months of drug discontinuation, although may rarely persist for up to 2 years. Dose reduction, interruption or complete withdrawal is recommended, along with symptomatic treatment.

Severe (grade 3–4) neuropathy has been reported in as many as 30% of patients receiving twice-weekly intravenous bortezomib, compared with fewer than 5% with protocols using weekly subcutaneous treatment; nevertheless, 40% of patients still experience emergent mild neuropathy on treatment. Close monitoring for neuropathy is therefore essential during bortezomib treatment.

Management of peripheral neuropathy. Patients should be evaluated for common causes of peripheral neuropathy and other distinct syndromes associated with M protein. Neurotoxic drug treatments are contraindicated in patients with moderate-to-severe neuropathy, and should be used with caution in patients with pre-existing mild peripheral neuropathy. Treatment-induced peripheral neuropathy should be closely monitored and managed as described above.[2]

Neuropathic pain responds poorly to standard analgesia. Opioids can be helpful in patients with mild neuropathy, together with reduction or withdrawal of the responsible agent. Patients with persistent neuropathy need additional pain modulators such as calcium-channel inhibitors, serotonin- and norepinephrine-reuptake inhibitors or sodium-channel-blocking agents; consultation with a pain specialist can be helpful.

Gabapentin or pregabalin, used regularly with opioids, can control neuropathic pain effectively in a significant proportion of patients. Close monitoring for adverse effects and dependence is required, particularly when regular opiates are used.

Use of topical analgesia with capsaicin cream, menthol, emollients and lidocaine plasters, can also be useful.

Hemostasis and thrombosis

The incidence of venous thromboembolism (VTE) in patients with MM varies widely but is estimated to be 5–10%. A recent retrospective study reported the incidence of deep vein thrombosis to be 8.7 per 1000 in patients with MM and 3.1 per 1000 in patients with MGUS, compared with 0.9 per 1000 in patients without plasma cell disorders. Various factors are thought to influence the development of VTE in patients with MM, including:

- postsurgical immobility
- use of central venous catheters
- pre-existing or acquired abnormalities in clotting factor production or platelet function
- treatment with anti-angiogenic (i.e. immunomodulatory) agents (e.g. thalidomide, lenalidomide or pomalidomide).

Patients with MM and related disorders are also at increased risk of arterial thrombosis.

One of the most important risk factors for the development of VTE in patients with MM is the type of chemotherapy used. The risk appears to be particularly high when immunomodulatory agents are combined with anthracyclines for the treatment of newly diagnosed disease. Combinations including thalidomide, lenalidomide or pomalidomide with pulsed dexamethasone, alkylating agents, or both, are associated with an intermediate risk, whereas the use of the same regimens for relapsed and refractory multiple myeloma (RRMM) seems to be associated with the lowest risk.

The risk of VTE is thought to be due to a reduction in thrombomodulin levels, a receptor responsible for binding to thrombin and converting it from a procoagulant to an anticoagulant enzyme. Thalidomide may also have an additional coagulant effect due to altered expression of protease-activated receptor 1 (PAR-1) at sites of endothelial injury; this may explain findings of hypercoagulability in patients treated with chemotherapy followed by thalidomide. An increase in VTE risk has also been observed in patients receiving dexamethasone, linked to endothelial damage, thereby predisposing to clotting.

Both venous and arterial thrombosis are associated with significant morbidity in patients with MM, and are associated with decreased survival. Prevention of thrombosis is therefore imperative. Guidelines from the International Myeloma Working Group (IMWG) for thrombosis risk assessment in patients with MM receiving therapy (Table 12.3) are widely used for risk stratification. They take into account patient-related factors such as previous VTE and obesity, myeloma-related factors such as plasma hyperviscosity and disease burden, and treatment-related factors such as the use of high-dose steroids. In previously untreated patients with low VTE risk, acetylsalicylic acid (ASA; aspirin) is an effective and less expensive alternative to thromboprophylaxis with low molecular weight heparins (LMWHs). VTE in patients receiving thromboprophylaxis should be managed according to local treatment guidelines.[3]

TABLE 12.3

Guidelines for VTE prophylaxis in patients with multiple myeloma receiving immunomodulatory agents

Individual risk factors
- Obesity (BMI ≥ 30 kg/m^2)
- Previous venous thromboembolism
- Central venous catheter or pacemaker
- Chronic renal disease (creatinine clearance < 40 mL/minute)
- Diabetes mellitus
- Medications (e.g. erythropoietin, estrogens)
- Immobility
- General surgery
- Trauma (major or lower extremity)
- Blood clotting disorders

Treatment-related risk factors
- High-dose dexamethasone (≥ 480 mg/month or 120 mg/week)
- Doxorubicin
- Combination chemotherapy

Number of risk factors	Prophylaxis
0–1	ASA, 81–325 mg daily
≥ 2	LMWH (enoxaparin 40 mg sc daily, or equivalent)

ASA, acetylsalicylic acid (aspirin); BMI, body mass index; LMWH, low molecular weight heparin; sc subcutaneous; VTE, venous thromboembolism.
Source: International Myeloma Working Group.

Coagulopathy

Bleeding is rare in MM but can result from thrombocytopenia secondary to disease progression, renal failure, infection or treatment toxicity. Paraproteinemia in MM can cause bleeding due to:
- acquired von Willebrand's disease
- plasma hyperviscosity
- platelet dysfunction

- factor X deficiency
- fibrin polymerization defects
- hyperfibrinolysis or circulating heparin-like anticoagulants
- associated AL amyloidosis.

Reducing plasma paraprotein can improve hemorrhagic manifestations, and platelet counts should be closely monitored on therapy. Recombinant factor VIIa and splenectomy have been reported to be successful in the management of bleeding in patients with factor X deficiency due to AL amyloidosis. There is lack of consensus on the management of acquired von Willebrand's disease in MM: bleeding episodes have been managed with variable success with desmopressin (producing at best a transient response), intravenous immunoglobulin infusions or factor VIII/von Willebrand factor concentrates. Management of bleeding in patients with MM needs to be individualized; discussion with a specialist in hemostasis is recommended.

Fatigue

Fatigue is reported by a significant proportion of patients with MM. It is often a major cause of poor quality of life but is largely under-recognized by healthcare professionals. Fatigue is usually multifactorial: treatable causes include anemia, renal impairment, treatment with analgesics and anti-myeloma therapies, low testosterone, and secretion of cytokines as a result of the disease process. These causes should be addressed and drug treatment optimized in order to reduce fatigue. In addition, psychological causes of mental fatigue are common and should be explored by a specialist nurse in collaboration with a psychologist.

Patients often have poor calorie intake, which should be addressed with the assistance of a dietitian; calorie supplementation with high-calorie energy drinks should be encouraged. Anti-myeloma drugs can cause loss of taste and appetite, which should be identified early. Patients are often poorly hydrated; where appropriate, they should be encouraged to drink up to 3 liters of fluid daily (provided that renal function is not impaired).

Drug-related symptoms such as neuropathy, nocturia, bowel disturbances and bone pain can compromise sleep. It is important to address these symptoms, encourage activity and advise against napping during the day; in rare circumstances, medications to promote sleep should be considered. There is robust evidence that aerobic exercise improves mood and physical functioning; physical activity should be encouraged after periods of hospitalization, particularly for stem cell transplantation.

Patients should be referred to general or spinal physiotherapy services as appropriate, and linked to local support groups and exercise programs in the community (see Useful resources, pages 150–1).

Managing the last 6 months of life

It is important for healthcare teams to recognize a patient with rapidly progressing and untreatable disease, as death is likely within 6 months. Usually this is evident from the presence of a refractory relapse, confirmed by lack of response to therapy, low blood counts and ongoing disease-related symptoms.

At this point, the myeloma team should consider referring the patient to a palliative care team, even if there are no significant symptoms necessitating assistance, as this allows team and patient to become acquainted. A holistic needs assessment at this point can highlight new problems and issues other than symptoms, such as psychosocial difficulties, existential concerns and decisions about future care.

Careful consideration is required about the use of further therapy, entry into early-stage experimental therapy trials, or withdrawal of anti-myeloma drugs. Patients may find this discussion uncomfortable, and it is therefore essential that family members or carers are involved (with the patient's consent).

Patients can choose to continue active therapy with symptomatic support, and this should be recognized and patients treated appropriately. Conversely, for patients who choose a minimalistic approach to anti-myeloma therapy, discussion of the patient's preferences for future care is warranted, including care towards the end of life and the use of life-maintaining treatments.

End-of-life care focuses on the patient's priorities in their last few days. At this stage, performance status declines significantly, with the onset of profound anorexia, extreme fatigue and sometimes reduced levels of consciousness. Pain and other symptoms may become refractory to previously optimal management, in which case support from the palliative care team should be sought. Family carers and dependents have their own needs at this stage, which should be addressed. Patients and carers may prefer to stay in hospital or in a hospice, or occasionally spend the last days at home.

Key points – supportive care

- Supportive care requirements for patients with multiple myeloma (MM) are related to disease activity, complications from anti-myeloma therapy and disease progression.
- Thalidomide and bortezomib both cause varying degrees of neuropathy in patients with MM.
- Infection is one of the frequent causes of early death in patients with MM.
- Patients with refractory relapses with few further treatment options should be jointly managed with a palliative care team.

References

1. Colson K. Treatment-related symptom management in patients with multiple myeloma: a review. *Support Care Cancer* 2015;23: 1431–45.

2. Koeppen S. Treatment of multiple myeloma: thalidomide-, bortezomib-, and lenalidomide-induced peripheral neuropathy. *Oncol Res Treat* 2014;37:506–13.

3. Larocca A, Cavallo F, Bringhen S et al. Aspirin or enoxaparin thromboprophylaxis for patients with newly diagnosed multiple myeloma treated with lenalidomide. *Blood* 2012;119:933–9.

4. Cousins MJ, Gallagher RM. *Fast Facts: Chronic and Cancer Pain*, 4th edn. Oxford: Health Press, 2017.

Useful resources

UK

Leukaemia and Lymphoma Research
Tel: +44 (0)20 7504 2200
www.leukaemialymphomaresearch.org.uk

London Cancer Alliance
Tel: +44 (0)20 7808 2644
lca.information@nhs.net
www.londoncanceralliance.nhs.uk

Macmillan Cancer Support
Helpline: 0808 808 00 00
Overseas helpline:
+44 (0)20 7091 2230
Tel: +44 (0)20 7840 7840
www.macmillan.org.uk

Myeloma UK
Infoline: 0800 980 3332
Tel: +44 (0) 0131 557 3332
www.myeloma.org.uk and
www.myelomatv.org.uk
(Myeloma TV)

National Amyloidosis Centre
Tel: +44 (0)20 7433 2725
www.ucl.ac.uk/amyloidosis/nac

UK Myeloma Forum
www.ukmf.org.uk

USA

Amyloidosis Foundation
Tel: +1 877 269 5643
www.amyloidosis.org

Leukemia and Lymphoma Society
Tel: +1 914 949 5213
Infoline: 1 800 955 4572
www.lls.org

Multiple Myeloma Research Foundation
Tel: +1 203 229 0464
info@themmrf.org
www.themmrf.org

The Binding Site
Toll-free: 1 800 633 4484
info@thebindingsite.com
www.thebindingsite.com/hematology

The Myeloma Beacon
info@myelomabeacon.com
www.myelomabeacon.com

International

Amyloidosis Australia
Tel: +61 (0)3 9001 9312
info@amyloidosis.com.au
www.amyloidosis.com.au

International Myeloma Foundation
Hotline: 1 800 452 2873
Infoline: +1 818 487 7455
TheIMF@myeloma.org
www.myeloma.org

International Waldenstrom's Macroglobulinemia Foundation
Tel: +1 941 927 4963
www.iwmf.com

Leukaemia and Blood Cancer New Zealand
Toll-free: 0800 15 10 15
Tel: +64 (0)9 638 3556
info@leukaemia.org.nz
www.leukaemia.org.nz

Myeloma Australia
Toll-Free: 1800 693 566
Tel: +61 03 9428 7444
www.myeloma.org.au

Myeloma Canada
Toll-free: 1 888 798 5771
Tel: +1 514 421 2242
contact@myeloma.ca
www.myelomacanada.ca

Myeloma Euronet
Tel: +49 (0) 6142 / 3 22 40
buero@lhrm.de
myelom-gruppe.lhrm.de

Nordic Myeloma Study Group
www.nordic-myeloma.org

Index

acetaminophen 139
African Americans 10–11, 16
age
  epidemiology 7–9, 15, 110
  organ dysfunction 17–18
  treatment 59, 64–5, 71–2, 129
AL amyloidosis 104, 108–21, 147
  localized 111–12, 118
  and MGUS 20, 111
albumin 40, 113
alkaline phosphatase 37, 120
alkylating agents 33, 55, 62, 106, 130, 135
  see also melphalan
allogeneic SCT 67, 73–4, 132
amyloidosis see AL amyloidosis
anakinra 22
analgesia 103, 139–40, 144
anemia 18, 36, 137–8
autologous stem cell transplantation (ASCT) 59, 63, 67, 71–3, 106, 118, 134, 140
  ineligible patients 64–5, 118–19, 135
autonomic neuropathy 113, 142, 143

B cells 28–31
  see also plasma cells
bacterial infections 21, 140
Bence Jones protein 39
bendamustine 106
β2-microglobulin 39
Bing–Neel syndrome 126–7
biomarkers
  amyloidosis 113, 116, 117, 119
  bone disease 22, 37, 101

biomarkers *continued*
  MGUS 16
  MM 36–9
  plasmacytoma 123–4
  POEMS syndrome 132, 134
  WM 128
bisphosphonates 102, 139
black ethnicity 10–11, 16
blood films 37
bone disease 98–103, 106
  biomarkers 22, 37, 101
  imaging 41–2, 99, 100–1
  in MGUS 21, 22
  osteoporosis 17, 21, 22, 99
  pain 99, 100, 103, 122, 138–40
  plasmacytoma 122
bone marrow
  examination 19, 39–41, 48, 116, 124, 134
  microenvironment 32–3, 100
bortezomib
  AL amyloidosis 118
  conditioning therapy 71
  induction therapy 58, 60–1, 62, 65, 66, 72
  mode of action 33
  neuropathy 143
  renal disease 105, 106
  RRMM 81, 86–7, 90–1
BRAF mutations 54

cardiac amyloidosis 113, 116, 116–17, 119, 120
carfilzomib 33, 62, 88–90
cast nephropathy 104
cellular therapies 74–5
chimeric antigen receptor T cells (CART) 74–5
chromosomal abnormalities 32, 43, 51–4, 81, 111
clinical presentation *see* signs and symptoms

clonal tiding 55–6
coagulopathy 113–14, 146–7
conditioning therapy 71
CRAB criteria 16, 25, 57
cryoglobulins 22, 127
CT (computed tomography) 42, 101, 124
cytogenetics 51–4
cytokines 32–3, 100

daratumumab 93
dendritic cell vaccines 75
denosumab 102
dental health 102
dermopathy 22–3, 132
dexamethasone
  adverse effects 140, 145
  induction therapy 59–62, 64–5, 72, 105
  POEMS syndrome 135
  RRMM 80, 81, 88, 91, 92, 93
diagnosis
  AL amyloidosis 114–17
  bone disease 41–2, 98–9, 100–1
  MGUS 16–18
  MM 35–42, 49
  plasmacytoma 123–4
  POEMS syndrome 132–4
  renal disease 37, 39, 104
  smoldering myeloma 23, 25
  WM 127–8
diarrhea 81
diet 147

elderly patients 64–5, 72, 129
electrophoresis 38
elotuzumab 92
end-of-life care 148–9
end organ damage 16, 17–18
  in AL amyloidosis 109, 112–13, 116–17

Index

environmental risk factors 11, 16
epidemiology
 AL amyloidosis 110
 MGUS 14–16
 MM 7–12
 smoldering myeloma 23
 WM 126
erythropoietin 138
ethnicity 10–11, 16
etiology 7–12, 16
exercise 148

family history 11, 126
fatigue 147–8
flow cytometry 19, 40, 46, 116, 128
fludarabine 130
fluid intake 147
fluorescence in situ hybridization (FISH) 51–4
fractures 21, 22, 99, 100, 101, 103, 122, 141
free light chains (FLCs) 30
 AL amyloidosis 109, 111, 116, 119
 and diagnosis 39, 104, 116
 light-chain MGUS 17
 progression to MM 19, 24, 25, 124
 RRMM 79
 and treatment 105, 119
fungal infections 140

gabapentin 144
gastrointestinal amyloidosis 113, 119
gender 9–10, 15
gene expression profiling 43–4, 54
genetics
 amyloidosis 111, 114
 assessment methods 51–5
 and choice of therapy 53, 54–6, 81
 MM/MGUS 10–11, 20, 31–2
 prognostic markers 43, 51, 54
 after treatment 55–6
 WM 127

hematological disorders
 anemia 18, 36, 137–8
 coagulopathy 113–14, 146–7
 thrombosis 21, 144–6
hepatic amyloidosis 113, 117, 120
herpes viruses 140–1
high-risk patients
 identification 23, 43, 44–5, 53, 54
 treatment 45, 65–7, 73
histone deacetylase (HDAC) inhibitors 90–2
HIV/AIDS 12
hypercalcemia 18, 37, 105
hyperparathyroidism 18, 37

ibrutinib 130–1
imaging
 AL amyloidosis 116, 117
 diagnosis 16, 18, 25, 41–2, 99, 100–1
 monitoring 46, 50
 plasmacytoma 123, 124
 POEMS syndrome 134
immunodeficiency 12, 21, 140
immunofixation 37–8, 116
immunoglobulins 30
 AL amyloidosis 109, 111, 116, 119
 diagnostic tests 37–9, 79
 MGUS 14, 17, 19, 24
 plasmacytoma 123–4
 POEMS syndrome 134
 renal damage 104, 105
 response to treatment 46
immunohistochemistry 40, 114
immunomodulatory drugs (ImiD)
 adverse effects 81, 143, 145
 AL amyloidosis 118–19
 induction therapy 59–62, 64–6, 72
 mode of action 33–4
 POEMS syndrome 135
 RRMM 80–1, 82–5

immunophenotyping 19, 40, 46, 116, 128
immunotherapy 74–5, 92–5, 102, 130
incidence 7, 9–10, 14, 110, 126
induction therapy 57–68, 72–3, 105
infections 12, 21, 140–1
interleukin-6 (IL-6) 32–3
International Myeloma Working Group (IMWG)
 MGUS 16, 20
 MM 25, 44, 49, 57, 66–7, 79
 thrombosis risk 145–6
isatuximb 93–4
ixazomib 33, 65, 90

karyotype 51, 52
kidney disease see renal disease
KRAS mutations 31, 54

lactate dehydrogenase 37, 44
lenalidomide 60, 65, 67, 72, 80–1, 82–3, 135
lifestyle measures 102, 147–8
light chains see free light chains (FLCs)
liver amyloidosis 113, 117, 120
liver function tests 37

M protein 14, 17, 31, 38, 46, 79, 104
macroglossia 113
management see treatment
melphalan 58, 64, 71, 72, 118, 134, 135
men 9–10, 15
minimal residual disease 48–50, 56
monitoring
 AL amyloidosis 119
 MGUS 23, 24
 MM 45–50
 plasmacytoma 124–5
 POEMS syndrome 135

153

monoclonal antibodies, therapeutic 74, 92–5, 102, 130
monoclonal gammopathy of undetermined significance (MGUS) 11, 12, 14–21, 23, 26–7, 31
and AL amyloidosis 20, 111
dermopathy 22–3
MGRS 21–2, 105–6
MGSS 21, 22
neuropathy 22, 141
and WM 126
monoclonal immunoglobulin deposition disease (MIDD) 104
morphine 139
mortality rates 7, 9, 10
MRI (magnetic resonance imaging) 25, 42, 46, 101, 117, 124
mutational analysis 54–5
Myd88 gene 20, 127
myeloid malignancies 21

nephrotic syndrome 113
neuropathy 141–4
amyloidosis 113, 117, 120
MGUS 22, 141
POEMS syndrome 132, 136
WM 126–7
NK cell-based infusions 74
non-Hodgkin lymphoma 20, 116
NSAIDs 139
NT-proBNP 115, 117

obesity 11
opioids 139–40, 144
oprozomib 90
orthostatic hypotension 119
osteolytic disease *see* bone disease
osteoporosis 17, 21, 22, 99
oxycodone 139

p53 deletion 61, 127
pain
bone 99, 100, 103, 122, 138–40
neuropathic 144
palliative care 103, 129, 148–9
pamidronate 102
panobinostat 91–2
paracetamol 139
paraprotein (M protein) 14, 17, 31, 38, 46, 79, 104
parathyroid disease 18, 37
pathophysiology
AL amyloidosis 109, 111
bone disease 100
kidney disease 104
MM/MGUS 28–34
WM 127
pembrolizumab 94–5
performance status 35, 64, 72, 98, 129, 149
personalized medicine 53, 55–6
PET-CT (positron emission tomography-CT) 42, 124
physiotherapy 136, 148
plasma cells 15, 17, 28, 31–3, 40–1
normal development 28–31
plasma exchange 105, 129
plasma hyperviscosity 129
plasmacytoma 122–6
POEMS syndrome 22, 132–5
pomalidomide 67, 81, 84–5
prednisone 64
pregabalin 144
prevalence 7, 14–16
primary refractory MM 63, 79
prognosis 37, 42–5
AL amyloidosis 117
genetics 43, 51, 54
WM 129
progression
from MGUS 18–20
from plasmacytoma 124
from smoldering myeloma 25–6

proteasome inhibitors
AL amyloidosis 118
conditioning therapy 71
induction therapy 59–62, 64–6, 67, 72
mode of action 33
neuropathy 143
renal disease 105, 106
RRMM 81, 86–91

radiation as a risk factor 11, 14
radiography 16, 41, 99, 100–1, 123
radioscintigraphy 42, 116, 117
radiotherapy 103, 125–6, 134
RANK ligand 100, 102
rasburicase 105
red blood cells 36
referral, of MGUS 23, 24
relapsed AL amyloidosis 119
relapsed and refractory MM (RRMM) 48, 54, 63, 78–95
relapsed WM 131
renal biopsy 39, 104
renal disease 18, 37, 39, 103–6
amyloidosis 104, 113, 117, 119, 120
MGRS 21–2, 105–6
treatment 104–6, 119
renal transplantation 106, 119
response assessment 46, 47–8
risk factors
for MM 7–12
for thrombosis 146
for WM 126
risk of progression
from MGUS 18–20
from plasmacytoma 124
from smoldering myeloma 25–6
risk stratification 43–5, 51, 54
rituximab 130
Rouleaux formations 37

Schnitzler's syndrome 22
serum amyloid P
  component (SAP) 116
serum FLCs (sFLCs) *see*
  free light chains
sex 9–10, 15
signs and symptoms
  AL amyloidosis 112–14
  bone disease 98–100
  MM 35
  neuropathy 142
  plasmacytoma 122–3
  POEMS syndrome 132,
    133
  WM 126–7
skin conditions 22–3, 132
SLiM CRAB criteria 25, 57
smoldering myeloma 15,
  23–6, 59
spinal disease 98–9, 100,
  101, 102, 103, 122, 141
staging 40, 42–3
  AL amyloidosis 117
stem cell transplantation
  allogeneic 67, 73–4, 132
  autologous 59, 63, 67,
    71–3, 106, 118, 134, 140
steroids *see*
  dexamethasone
supportive care 102, 119,
  136, 137–49
  analgesia 103, 139–40,
    144
survival rates 7, 40, 44,
  117, 129

thalidomide 33–4, 66, 72,
  80, 118–19, 143, 145
thrombocytopenia 146
thrombosis 21, 144–6
tongue enlargement 113
tramadol 139
treatment
  AL amyloidosis 117–19
  allo-SCT 67, 73–4, 132
  ASCT 59, 63, 67, 71–3,
    106, 118, 134, 140
  assessment of 45–50,
    55–6, 130
  bone disease 102–3,
    139–40
  cellular therapies 74–5
  conditioning therapy 71
  end-of-life 148–9
  high-risk patients 45,
    65–7, 73
  induction therapy 57–68,
    72–3, 105
  maintenance therapy 53,
    66
  modes of action of drugs
    33–4, 90
  plasmacytoma 125–6
  POEMS syndrome 134–6
  renal disease 104–6, 119
  RRMM 54, 63, 78–95
  smoldering myeloma 25,
    59
  supportive care 102, 119,
    136, 137–49

treatment *continued*
  transplant-ineligible
    patients 64–5, 118–19,
    135
  WM 128–32
troponin T 117

urinary tests 39, 113, 116

vaccines 75
venous thromboembolism
  (VTE) 21, 144–6
vertebral disease 98–9,
  100, 101, 102, 103, 122,
  141
viral infections 12, 21,
  140–1
vitamin D 102
von Willebrand's disease,
  acquired 147
vorinostat 91

Waldenström's
  macroglobulinemia
  (WM) 20, 126–32
women 9–10, 15

X-rays 16, 41, 99, 100–1,
  123

zoledronic acid 102

Notes

Notes

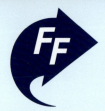

Fast Facts – the ultimate medical handbook series covers over 70 topics, including:

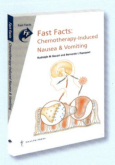
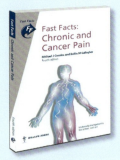
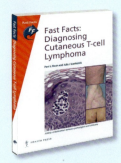
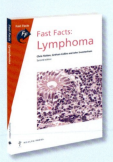
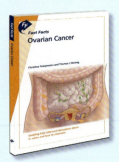
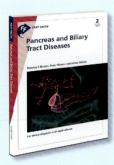

FastTest

You've read the book ... now test yourself with key questions from the authors

- Go to the FastTest for this title **FREE** at **fastfacts.com**
- Approximate time **10 minutes**
- For best retention of the key issues, try taking the FastTest before and after reading

And for your patients...

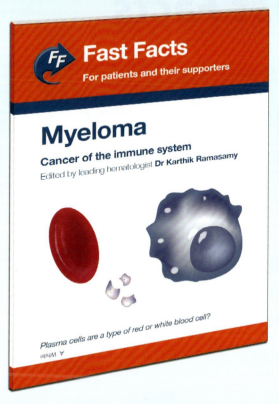

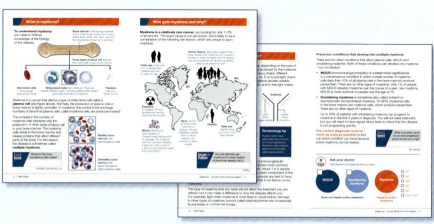

fastfacts.com

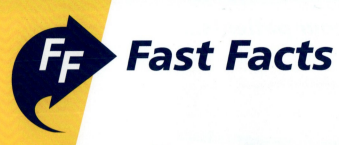

Fast Facts

Reading for results
(and tests worth taking)

With so much to read these days, you need to be selective ...

Was this Fast Facts well worth reading?

Has it helped you make good health decisions?

Did it trigger new ideas you'd like to explore?

If so, please post them in the comments box on the relevant page on **www.fastfacts.com**, and check out fellow readers' insights while you're there.

This is also the place to leave questions for the authors' consideration, and to spend 10 minutes on the free **FastTest** to ensure those key points really sunk in, and that you are set to apply them – **result!**

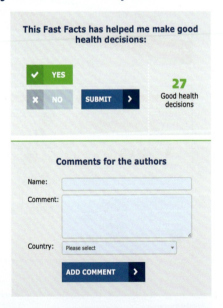

fastfacts.com